THE
CORONER'S INVESTIGATOR'S
HANDBOOK

2ND EDITION

MRS ALI WARNER MSC

Published by:-
ECRI Europe
Weltech Centre
Ridgeway
Welwyn Garden City
Herts
AL7 2AA
United Kingdom

Tel: +44 (0)1707 871511
Fax: +44 (0)1707 393138
E-mail: info@ecri.org.uk
Web: www.ecri.org

Second publication 2009
First published 2005

ISBN 0-9549718-1-7

FOREWORD
BY DR JAMES ADELEY
HM CORONER PRESTON AND WEST LANCASHIRE

In the last ten years the work of the Coroner's Service has expanded both in terms of the issues with which it is required to deal and the complexity of the investigations required. The scope of the inquest has been broadened by the rapid development of Human Rights Act 1998 by the courts requiring detailed investigations. The areas of investigation where interest is most concentrated include healthcare related deaths where there is the possibility of medical manslaughter, a failure of NHS systems to prevent patients' deaths and detention of patients under the Mental Heath Acts as well as the perennial problem of deaths in state custody. Other legislation affecting the Coroner's Service is the Human Tissue Act 2004 and Corporate Manslaughter Act 2007. At the current time the Coroner's and Justice Bill is moving through the legislative process and, in whatever form it is enacted, will resolve some difficulties and create other challenges.

At the sharp end of this period of change is the Coroner's Staff and particularly the Coroner's Forensic Investigator. It has always been my view that the adequacy of any inquest and the satisfaction of the bereaved family depend upon the skills base and knowledge of the investigator involved. Consequently, the first edition of this book was required reading for any investigator in my jurisdiction.

The new edition of Mrs Warner's book builds extensively on the success of the first edition, which is of itself no mean feat. This second edition retains its ease of reading but incorporates additional commentary on healthcare deaths, investigations which involve consideration of the requirements of human rights, specialists who may be able to assist in identification, information about organisations able to assist in healthcare investigations and a plethora of other updated information.

I would warmly recommend this book to investigators, to either teach or improve the broad range of skills an investigator is now required to possess.

I would also recommend any newly appointed Assistant Deputy Coroner read this book if they wish to know the range of questions that may be asked in respect of various deaths.

INTRODUCTION

This book provides guidance to those who investigate deaths on behalf of Her Majesty's Coroners. It is unique in its approach and understanding of the requirements of Coroners. There is as yet, no other book that considers the investigation of deaths from the perspective of a Coroner's Investigator – as opposed to the forensic criminal perspective.

The investigation of death is an important marker within society. Death affects everyone as they journey through their own life, somehow or other. A society can be classified according to the systems it has in place for dealing with death as it can for birth, health and other life experiences.

"Most people are pleased to live in a society in which there is a thorough system of judicially investigating unnatural deaths. Imagine living in a society in which unnatural deaths... were not investigated with a view to finding out the identity of the deceased, and how, when and where the death occurred. Such a system would allow all sorts of sinister conduct and cover-ups." Slapper (2003)

This book is written to assist the death scene investigator, as opposed to a forensic specialist who forms part of the criminal process. It seems likely that Coroner's Officers will increasingly carry out this role. Many Coroner's Officers do not have experience in this area and some foundations are provided herein.

The investigation of deaths on behalf of Coroners currently varies from one jurisdiction to another, as to who carries out the investigation, to what depth enquiries are made, and what expertise the Investigator has. Additionally each Coroner has different expectations:

"Unfortunately the great difficulty in writing anything about coroners is the variation in both practice and procedure from jurisdiction to jurisdiction." Dorries (1999)

"There are more than 120 coroners and probably almost as many (correct) (sic) ways of approaching an inquest." (Dorries 2004)

Other factors affecting the approach to, and standard of, death investigation may include who actually carries it out. The investigator may be a police officer - as currently in some areas - or a dedicated Coroner's Officer / Investigator (see Chapter 1 for further discussion on the title of this role).

In the introduction to the government's paper: "Reforming the Coroner and Death Certification Service A Position Paper" (2004) the Home Secretary stated:

"The new coronial system we propose must be:
Consistent – a uniform service across England and Wales, and Northern Ireland, with unified high standards of performance." (op cit)

The investigation of a death with an inquest in mind is not required to be dealt with in the same way as those that are "suspicious", requiring a full police forensic investigation. However it does require thoroughness to obtain the best possible evidence for the Coroner.

In offering a general framework that can be applied to all "non-criminal" scenes, this book seeks to encourage individuality that leads to innovation, whilst remaining within robust parameters. In offering specific suggestions and individual checklists for specific types of death, the aim is to assist the Coroner's Investigator in providing a professional service to Coroners, families, the courts and society. The most commonly encountered deaths are considered in depth in subsequent chapters.

Much of this book is based upon the practical experience of investigating deaths on behalf of a Coroner with exacting and high standards, in an environment where the police resources are freed up to carry out their many other duties by the Coroner's Officers carrying out a full investigative function where appropriate.

Where the term "family" is used it is with an acknowledgment that there is as yet no clearly defined adequate term to cover "next of kin", "partner", "significant other" to accurately reflect the wider group of people who may be involved with a deceased. The Human Tissue Act 2004 has taken steps to address this very issue, providing a "hierarchy of next of kin". Rather than explain in every instance, it is assumed that "family" is used in the widest possible sense of the word.

Reference is made throughout to various documents that have already started to impact on the world of Coroners and their Investigators and are likely to do so more within the next five to ten years. These are (in no particular order):

The Report on the Provision of Coroner's Officers (2002); hereinafter referred to as the HOWP Report (2002), where HOWP stands for Home Office Working Party.

Reforming the Coroner and Death Certification Service A Position Paper (March 2004) already cited above; hereinafter referred to as the government's position paper (2004).

The Shipman Inquiry Third Report Death Certification and the Investigation of Deaths by Coroners (July 2003); hereinafter referred to as the Shipman Inquiry Report (2003).

Coroner Reform and Additional Medical Advice (August 2007); hereinafter referred to as the Ministry of Justice (MoJ) discussion document 2007.

Statutory Duty for Doctors and other Public Service Personnel to Report Deaths to the Coroner (July 2007); hereinafter referred to as the MoJ consultation paper 2007.

Coroner Reform: The Government's Draft Bill Improving death investigation in England and Wales (June 2006); hereinafter referred to as the draft Coroner's Reform Bill 2006.

Coroners and Justice Bill (laid before Parliament on 14/1/2009).

Coroners and Justice Act 2009 (due to receive Royal Assent in 2009).

Death Certification and Investigation in England, Wales and Northern Ireland The Report of a Fundamental Review (2003); hereinafter referred to as the Fundamental Review Report 2003.

Consultation on Improving the Process of Death Certification (July 2007); hereinafter referred to as the Department of Health (DH) consultation paper 2007.

Improving the Process of Death Certification in England and Wales: Overview of Programme (November 2008); hereinafter referred to as the Department of Health programme overview paper 2008.

It is hard to anticipate the precise changes that will affect the coronial system with a high degree of accuracy at the time of going to press. I have taken the approach of "a balance of probabilities" that Coroner's Officers will recognise well.

Chapter 1 considers that the Coroner will have a dedicated team of Investigators working on his behalf, separate from the police. Whether that is the case or not, the topics remain valid for any variety of situations that may arise.

Chapters 2 – 12 consider specific investigations needed by the Coroner without being specific as to who does the investigation – be that a police officer, Coroner's Officer, Coroner's Investigator (CI) or other agency.

Chapters 13 – 17 consider more generic matters.

On matters of grammar and terminology:

To avoid complication of gender, he is taken to mean both he and she etc.

Her Majesty's Coroner will be referred to throughout as Coroner rather than HM Coroner. This is for ease and does not in any way demean the importance of the office held.

The term Coroner is used in the most generic sense of the word within the parameters of the Coroners and Justice Bill. Schedule 3 Part 1 of this Bill refers to "senior coroner", "area coroner" and "assistant coroner". Schedule 3 Part 3 Paragraph 7 allows for area coroners or assistant coroners to "act" as coroner when a vacancy occurs and before a new appointment is made. Schedule 3 Part 3 Paragraph 8 allows for area coroners or assistant coroners to:

"perform any functions of the senior coroner for the area .... (a) during a period when that senior coroner is absent or unavailable; (b) at any other time, with the consent of that senior coroner".

As regards apostrophes: The legislation on Coroner's Act 1988 and Coroner's Rules 1984 is sometimes referred to with an apostrophe and sometimes without. I have adopted the convention used by Her Majesty's Stationery Office – the publishers of the legislation. Thus: Coroners Act 1988; Coroners Rules 1984; and the Coroners and Justice Act 2009

The Coroner's Officers Association (COA) took the view some years ago that most Coroner's Officers work to one Coroner and not more than one. Thus the possessive apostrophe appears before the "s", rather than after it. I have followed that convention. Where other sources are quoted, this is verbatim and accordingly the apostrophe may vary in location. Similarly Coroner and Coroner's Officers are accorded capital letters throughout – unless being quoted from another source.

ACKNOWLEDGMENTS

I would like to express my deep gratitude to each of the following for their help and guidance with sections of this work:

Senior Scenes of Crime Officer Brian Gilbert (Sussex Police); Inspector Gary Ancell (BTP); Mr Stuart McNab, HMCG; Mr Peter Dymond, MCA; Mr Hugh Fogarty, RNLI; Mr David Wright, West Yorkshire Police; Mr Simon Sampson, forensic odontologist; Mr David Watson (ECRI); the many colleagues who have answered my many and various questions.

I would particularly like to thank Dr James Adeley, HM Coroner Preston & West Lancashire; Mr Alan Craze, HM Coroner East Sussex; and Miss Joanna Pratt, Deputy Coroner East Sussex whose support and advice have been tremendous throughout.

My special thanks to my husband whose support is infallible and whose acceptance of the permanent presence of a computer (even on holiday), never wavered.

Any mistakes made are of course unintentional, but my own.

Mrs Ali Warner

CONTENTS

ACKNOWLEDGMENTS

INTRODUCTION

THE CORONER'S INVESTIGATOR'S HANDBOOK

CHAPTER 7 DEATHS THROUGH INTOXICATION

7.01 Alcohol Related Deaths

    7.01.1 Introduction

    7.01.2 Specific investigation guidelines - over and above the generic checklist

        7.01.2.1 The deceased

        7.01.2.2 The body

        7.01.2.3 The scene where found

        7.01.2.4 Circumstances

        7.01.2.5 Other considerations

        7.01.2.6 Actions

        7.01.2.7 Statements to be obtained

7.02 Drug Related Deaths

    7.02.1 Prescribed drugs

        7.02.1.1 Drugs chart

        7.02.1.2 The deceased

        7.02.1.3 The finder

        7.02.1.4 The body

        7.02.1.5 The scene where found

        7.02.1.6 Circumstances

        7.02.1.7 The event

        7.02.1.8 Other considerations

        7.02.1.9 Actions

        7.02.1.10 Additional statements

    7.02.2 Illegal drugs

        7.02.2.1 Offences

        7.02.2.2 Verdicts

        7.02.2.3 Previous history

        7.02.2.4 The deceased

        7.02.2.5 The finder

        7.02.2.6 The body

        7.02.2.7 The scene where found

        7.02.2.8 Circumstances

        7.02.2.9 The event

        7.02.2.10 The time

CHAPTER 15 THE CORONER'S INVESTIGATOR - OTHER ROLES

15.01 Introduction

15.02 CI administrator

15.03 CI family liaison

    15.03.1 Cause of death

    15.03.2 Death registration

    15.03.3 Tissue and / or organ retention

    15.03.4 Inquest procedures

    15.03.5 Return of property

15.04 CI public relations

15.05 CI court usher

    15.05.1 Difficulties with witnesses

    15.05.2 Jurors

CHAPTER 16 TRAINING

16.01 Introduction

16.02 Training for CIs and MEOs

16.03 Training for CIs

16.04 Training for the CI - statement taker & evidence gatherer

16.05 Training for the CI - administrator

16.06 Training for the CI - family liaison

16.07 Training for the CI - court usher role

CHAPTER 17 CORONER'S INVESTIGATORS' EQUIPMENT

17.01 Introduction

17.02 Medical record keeping

    17.02.1 Standardisation

17.03 Investigative records

    17.03.1 Introduction

    17.03.2 How does this apply to the CI?

    17.03.3 A multi-function log book

        17.03.3.1 Time recording

        17.03.3.2 Daily activity log

        17.03.3.3 Description of the deceased

1

THE CORONER'S INVESTIGATOR

1.01 Introduction

The terms Coroner's Officer and Coroner's Investigator are not defined and the role of a Coroner's Officer / Investigator in one Coroner's jurisdiction and under one employer still varies enormously to that in another jurisdiction and employer area.

The existence of Coroner's Officers has now been recognised within the Coroners and Justice Bill but the term is still not defined:

"The relevant authority for a coroner area ... must secure the provision of whatever officers and other staff are needed by the coroners for that area to carry out their functions." (Coroners and Justice Bill Paragraph 23)

The term 'Coroner's Officer' is mentioned again in Paragraph 32(2) of the Bill. The Coroners and Justice Bill has made no move towards standardisation of the role.

In this book, Coroner's Officers will henceforth be referred to as Coroner's Investigators (CIs) unless in a reference from elsewhere in which case the original terminology will be used.

It can be stated that there are two possible main roles for a Coroner's Investigator – medical and forensic.

1.02 The medical Coroner's Investigator (CI)

Following publication of the Draft Coroner Reform Bill in 2006 there was consultation with the Department of Health as to the provision of medical advice for Coroners in the future:

"seeking view on proposals to address weaknesses in the current system for certifying death which were identified by the Shipman Inquiry." (The Department of Health consultation paper 2007).

In this paper it was suggested that

"The Medical Certificate of Cause of Death (MCCD) should be completed by the medical practitioner responsible for the deceased person's care... . After completion, the MCCD should be passed to a Medical Examiner ... . If the medical practitioner is unable to complete an MCCD, or for example if the death is violent or unnatural or suspicious, the death should be reported to the Coroner. The Medical Examiner will scrutinise the MCCD and investigate as necessary.... It will include for example, looking at the deceased's medical records and the results of investigations, discussing the circumstances of the death with the doctor signing the MCCD and other clinicians involved in the deceased's care and, where necessary, with the family of the deceased. If the Medical Examiner is satisfied that all is in order, he or she will issue an authorisation to the family of the deceased to enable them to register the death and proceed to burial or cremation. If not satisfied, the Medical Examiner will have a duty to refer the case to the Coroner for further investigation and to inform the family that he or she has done so. In this situation, the Medical Examiner should provide a recommendation on whether or not a post-mortem examination is likely to provide relevant information beyond that which is available from other sources (although the final decision to order a postmortem will continue to remain with the Coroner)." (op cit 5.3 – 5.6)

In a written statement to the House of Commons the Parliamentary Under-Secretary of State for Justice Bridget Prentice MP wrote:

"The Coroners and Justice Bill mentioned in the Queen's Speech on 3 December will create the role of medical examiner. The Medical Examiner will examine all

deaths not requiring coronial post mortem or inquest...." Hansard 17/12/2008 column 121WS

The role of Medical Examiner (ME) is introduced in the Coroners and Justice Bill:

"Primary Care Trusts (in England) and Local Health Boards (in Wales) must appoint persons as medical examiners to discharge the functions conferred on medical examiners by or under this Chapter.
(2) Each Trust or Board must –
(a) appoint enough medical examiners, and make available enough funds and other resources, to enable those functions to be discharged in its area." (Coroners and Justice Bill Chapter 2 Paragraph 18)

It is easy to foresee that the role of the medical Coroner's Investigator will be introduced, albeit possibly with a different title such as Medical Examiner's Officer (MEO).

The Department of Health programme overview paper 2008 (op cit) makes specific reference to MEOs working in the ME's office.

The Medical Examiner (ME) will not have time to make all the necessary enquiries himself, and will need staff to carry out investigations on his behalf. Details of the functions and tasks and expectations of the ME are not fully covered in the Coroners and Justice Bill. However that Bill allows for subsequent Regulations to detail the minutiae.

In this book medical CIs will henceforth be referred to as MEOs unless in a reference from elsewhere in which case the original terminology will be used.

The Department of Health (DH) has issued a series of documents on the DH website on the process of death certification for the future. In November 2008 an update was issued with a clear diagram as to the proposed process for death certification of all deaths, whether or not referred to the Coroner's

Office. See the DH programme overview paper 2008 on the process of death certification (op cit). Visit also www.dh.gov.uk/deathcertification.

BBC Radio 4 broadcast a programme about Dr Shipman on 12th February 2009 in which Dame Janet Smith spoke. An article appeared on the BBC website in connection with that programme in which it was stated:

"In a BBC interview, Dame Janet Smith, who chaired the Harold Shipman Inquiry, criticised the system of death certification in England and Wales.... The Coroners and Justice Bill includes plans for the appointment of medical examiners who will scrutinise death certificates and liaise with coroners on any issues of concern.
Dame Janet welcomes some aspects of the new legislation, but has concerns about other parts which are "not so good".
She is encouraged by plans to modernise the coroner system. However, she says the new arrangements for death certification remain unknown, and will require secondary legislation, which may lead to further delays. Until the details are known, she says she cannot see how the system will work. In addition, she is worried about the status of the medical examiners.
"It is said that he or she will be independent, but I fear that that will be very difficult. I do not see how an employee of the primary care trust can be independent of the National Health Service," she said.
"I wanted that person to work alongside the coroner."" (www.bbc.co.uk)

The Coroners and Justice Bill Chapter 2 Paragraph 19 (1) k refers to enquiries being able to be made by:

"someone acting on behalf of a medical examiner"

It seems that many deaths will be referred to the ME's office in the first instance and may be finalised there, requiring no onward referral to the Coroner's Department: Coroners and Justice Bill Chapter 2 Paragraph 19 (1) (b)).

In other cases the MEO will refer the death on the Coroner: Coroners and

THE CORONER'S INVESTIGATOR

Justice Bill Chapter 2 Paragraph 19 (1) (f) (ii). See also the flow chart in the DH programme overview paper 2008 (op cit).

In some cases a cause of death may be such that referral to the Coroner's Office is obviously required and may pass straight to the CI from the "attending practitioner" and not through the ME's office at all: Coroners and Justice Bill Chapter 2 Paragraph 19 (1) (a) (ii). See also the flow chart in the DH programme overview paper 2008 (op cit).

The term "attending practitioner" is defined in the Coroners and Justice Bill:

"registered medical practitioner who attended the deceased before his or her death": (Coroners and Justice Bill Chapter 2 Paragraph 19 (1) (a))

It follows that the CI will have to have the medical knowledge that an MEO has, as well as an understanding of the process which has already been gone through before the case arrives in the Coroner's office.

The transfer of information may be as simple as transferring the papers from one desk to another in the same office; one office to another in the same building.

"Medical examiners and Coroners may be co-located" (The Department of Health consultation paper 2007 5.13)

However if the ME and Coroner and their staff are not co-located there is a possibility that information could be lost in the transfer process and systems will need to be put in place to minimise this risk. Considering the needs of the family of the bereaved there will be a need for speed of transfer without loss of accurate information.

1.03 The role of the MEO

The role of the MEO will in all probability mainly involve taking the basic details for completion of a sudden death form, or equivalent, as required by the ME. These will vary from area to area but will involve collecting all the details the ME and / or Coroner needs; medical details for the pathologist; and details that the Registrar of Births, Deaths and Marriages will need.

If the death is reported straight to the Coroner's Office then the CI will take the details themselves.

The Shipman Inquiry Report (2003) commented:

"Even if the autopsy is taking place in the hospital where the deceased died, the medical records are not always examined. Some coroners and their officers provide high quality information for pathologists and are prepared to make any further enquiries requested. However, others are less efficient. Coroner's officers may be office-bound, may have no investigative role and may be unable to identify or discover further information which could be of assistance to the pathologist." (op cit para 9.20)

Referral of a death does not always necessarily result in a post mortem examination and it will be the MEO or CI who will uncovers the information for the ME / Coroner to make the most appropriate decision.

Questions that will need to be answered include:

- What are the circumstances surrounding the death?
- What is the past medical history (PMH)?
- Is there an "attending practitioner" able to issue a certificate as to the cause of death – but who has not seen the deceased within the appropriate time period before death?
- Is a post mortem necessary to establish the cause of death?
- If so what is the family's view on a post mortem examination?
- Do they feel one is necessary? If so what is their rationale?

- Would they prefer there not to be a post mortem – if the doctor were able and allowed to issue a death certificate with authority from the Coroner?

Once these questions are answered the ME / Coroner is in a better position to decide whether a post mortem examination will be necessary or not.

In August 2007 the Ministry of Justice (MoJ) issued a discussion document on the possible way forward for the provision of future medical advice to the Coroner service.

"Evidence given to the Shipman Inquiry and Luce Review showed that a substantial number of decisions taken in coroners' offices are medically related and given that some of these decisions required a detailed depth of medical knowledge, both reports recommended that coroners and their officers would benefit from some further expert support in this area. This is not a reflection on the quality of personnel currently working in the service – but on the unique nature of the work straddling complex legal and medical issues." (Coroner Reform and Additional Medical Advice 2007 3.1)

1.03.1 Specific aspects of the role of MEO

In 2002 the Home Office attempted to categorise some of the various tasks and roles performed by Coroner's Officers across the country in the HOWP report 2002 (op cit). This document was produced by a working party, consisting of the Home Office (HO), the Coroners' Society, Association of Chief Police Officers (ACPO), the Metropolitan Police, the Coroner's Officers Association (COA), and the Local Government Association (LGA).

The HOWP report (2002) comments that the "medical" role of the Coroner's Officer mainly involves office-based telephone work. It requires an understanding of, and familiarity with, medical matters. It includes:

- *Receiving paperwork from police who attended the death (if relevant)*
- *Taking details by telephone from person reporting (if police not attended) and completing the sudden death form*

- *Establishing whether there is enough information to refer the matter to the Coroner or whether more needs to be gathered before the Coroner can decide whether a post mortem examination is necessary or not*
- *Liaise with family / friends / next of kin*
- *Liaison with hospital medical staff, hospital bereavement officers, GPs - to obtain further information*
- *Tracing ante-mortem samples if appropriate*
- *Ensuring accurate spelling of medical terminology*
- *Referral of the case to the Coroner for a decision as to the need for a post mortem examination or not*
- *Alerting mortuary staff to any relevant infectious diseases or other health hazard (if relevant)*
- *Liaison with Registrars of Births and Deaths and with crematoria as needed*

It seems likely that the role of MEO will be largely similar to the above.

In July 2008 the Ministry of Justice (MoJ) and Coroner's Officers Association (COA) conducted a survey of the duties and practices of Coroner's Officers and administrative staff in England and Wales. Officers and staff who participated in the survey have been provided with a summary of the results but these have not been made publicly available.

1.04 Requirements of the role of MEO

1.04.1 Knowledge

Good knowledge of basic anatomy and physiology, including all common medical terms is vital. If the MEO (or CI) does not have a medical background, there is a Fundamental Medicine Course for Coroner's Officers supplied by the Coroner's Officers Association (see also Chapter 16 on Training).

1.04.2 Understanding

The MEO needs an understanding of:

- The role of the "attending practitioner" in death certification in the current system
- The role of the ME
- The role of the Coroner
- Procedures in relation to surgery and medical treatments in hospital
- Medical terminology
- Healthcare organisational structure within the NHS, including the roles of the MHRA (Medicine and Healthcare products Regulatory Agency); the Care Quality Commission (CQC); the PCT (Primary Care Trust) and NHS Business Service Authority Dental Services Division (NHS BSA DSD), etc
- The role of pathology in establishing causes of death
- Causes of death (both natural and unnatural) and the requirements of the Registrar of Births and Deaths in relation to these

1.04.3 Skills

An ability to:

- Ask appropriate questions and establish whether the death needs immediate referral to the Coroner
- Establish whether the death is one that needs more medical investigation before the Coroner can make the best decision as to whether a post mortem is necessary
- Ask questions to establish whether there is there an infection that needs flagging to the mortuary staff
- Liaise with the police who attend the routine sudden deaths and help complete their paperwork
- Translate medical terminology into understandable terminology for families

1.05 The forensic Coroner's Investigator (CI)

Introduction

Forensic is defined in the Collins Concise English Dictionary as:

"Characteristic of or suitable for a law court, public debate or formal argument."

It can be seen therefore that the CI has a responsibility to provide the best possible evidence to the Coroner for a formal exposition and a public debate in a law court. This responsibility remains constant no matter who fulfils the role of the CI in each individual case. It may be a police officer, a police civilian or a dedicated CI not police employed. In some instances the investigative role may be performed by more than one person. In such instances, the handover points need to be carefully managed to ensure a seamless service and a seamless level of evidence and continuity. Some of these issues are considered in this chapter.

1.06 Deaths referred to the Coroner

Where a death is clearly going to require an inquest then it is unlikely to ever pass through the ME's office in the first place, and is more likely to be referred by the "attending practitioner" to the Coroner via the CI: see Coroners and Justice Bill Chapter 2 Paragraph 19 (1) (a) (ii). See also the flow chart on the DH website on the process of death certification (op cit).

All the relevant reports over the past few years have referred to lists of deaths reportable to the Coroner. In each case inquestable deaths are included in the list.

The government's position paper (2004) states:

*"We believe that there is real value in holding a judicial inquest. This allows the death to be publicly investigated by a local coroner in a court setting. Two types of death might be **referred to the coroner:** (sic) those from a list of reportable cases .... see sample list at Annex 2)." (op cit paragraph 39)*

Annex 2 includes:

"Any violent or traumatic death, including all deaths apparently from self-harm."

The MoJ consultation paper (2007) suggested a list of deaths where there would be a statutory duty on certain personnel to report deaths to the Coroner. In this consultation paper reference was made to such lists existing in other countries, and the list proposed in the Luce report.

The Coroners and Justice Bill does not provide a list of deaths which must be referred directly to the Coroner.

See also section 1.10 below.

The CI needs to be able to do all that the MEO can do. This is not only so that they can understand what enquiries have already been undertaken, where appropriate, but also so that when the death has not already been referred through the ME system, the CI can start with those very enquiries themselves.

1.07 Tissue and organ issues

1.07.1 Tissue and organ retention
The CI will need to discuss issues of tissue and organ retention by the pathologist on the Coroner's authority with the family:

● Why has it been necessary at all?
● What will happen?
● How long will it take for the results to come through?
● Can the tissues and organs be returned before the funeral?
● What other choices do they have regarding the tissue samples?
● Will there be any delay to the funeral?
● Will some samples need to be retained for longer periods? Why? How long?
● Can there be a separate funeral for the organs at a later date?

The Coroners (Amendment) Rules 2005 govern what the family must be told and what their options are regarding ultimate disposal. The issues of tissue and organ retention need to be addressed early and the CI is well placed to explain these to the family. See also the CPIA (1996) Code of Practice 2005 which sets out the period for which evidence must be retained in criminal investigations.

1.07.2 Tissue and organ donation

The CI is aware of when tissue donation may be suitable or not; what the potential problems are; what questions to ask the other professionals while they are available; and of the time limits involved. The CI can make the contact with the co-ordinator at the National Blood Service Tissue Services; ensure the body is appropriately labelled (there are special requirements of information over and above normal labelling); talk to the family within the time limits involved, still giving the family the time to consider carefully this valuable option without being pressurised. This is a valuable service to the public. See also section 1.08.5.2 below.

1.08 Which deaths and why?

To achieve the best possible evidence the CI will always want to attend the scene of a death or the location of a deceased in any death which will need an investigation on behalf of the Coroner. This is whether a public hearing (currently known as an inquest) will or will not eventually be required. The Coroner and the public need to be assured that there has been as full an investigation as possible.

Increasingly deaths in healthcare environments are being referred to the Coroner for investigation. The CI needs to have a good understanding of what medical records are available that should be obtained as part of their investigations on behalf of the Coroner, and how to obtain those records. (See also Chapters 9 - 12 on healthcare related deaths.)

The Shipman Inquiry Report (2003) commented:

"Even if the autopsy is taking place in the hospital where the deceased died, the medical records are not always examined. Some coroners and their officers provide

high quality information for pathologists and are prepared to make any further enquiries requested. However, others are less efficient. (op cit para 9.20)

In considering this important role for the CI it is worth considering the final goals:

1) The full investigation that the Coroner needs to have had carried out into any such death

2) The inquest itself. This is the public hearing into the investigations that have been carried out. The Coroner may decide not to publicly explore as much detail as the investigation has gathered.

1.08.1 Which scenes of death does a CI attend?

Simply – any, where there is a scene and where there will be or may be a subsequent investigation required.

In some cases it is apparent from the outset that an inquest investigation will need to take place e.g. death due to a road traffic collision. Such deaths are not regarded as "natural" deaths and an inquest will need to be held.

In others it is possible that an inquest hearing may need to take place - e.g. a decomposed body. This is because the cause of death is quite likely to be unascertainable – which always requires further investigation - enabled by the inquest investigative process.

It is far better for a CI to have attended a death and treated it as an inquestable death – only later to find that it was in fact due to natural causes and the attendance was unnecessary. The reverse scenario – to have not attended a death – and later wish to have done so, is a much worse position to be in, for the Coroner, the CI, the family of the deceased and the general public.

It is very important that someone trained in and knowledgeable of coronial ways, attends the scene and investigates the death thoroughly from the very beginning. The Coroner is much less able to decide whether a witness needs to attend in person or not to give evidence, if evidence is missing, was not gathered, or is no longer available. Every effort must be made to ensure that families and Coroners are not put in the embarrassing position of having to hold a public inquest hearing simply because a death was not properly investigated in the first place. This could mean that the Coroner would not be able to have a "full and fearless" enquiry without calling witnesses to give evidence in person at any inquest hearing.

1.08.2 The purpose of an inquest (being the public hearing)

Mr Michael Burgess, HM Coroner Surrey and former Secretary of the Coroners' Society, has suggested that quite apart from the reasons outlined in the often cited Jamieson case of 1993, the following is appropriate when considering the purpose of an inquest:

"An inquest provides live evidence, with sworn witnesses who can be questioned by the Coroner (and others). The evidence can be accepted or rejected and a decision can be made on the evidence heard. It is a 2 way dialogue in which the Coroner seeks to obtain evidence upon which he/she reaches decisions which are then communicated and explained." (Talk to new Coroners, Northampton April 2002)

Mr Christopher Dorries, HM Coroner South Yorkshire (West), said in a talk to the Coroner's Officers Association in June 2003 of inquests, that:

● the interests of society require an open investigation into a violent death

● the inquest should establish the true facts so far as possible and consider whether the initial investigation (by the police or some other authority) has in fact established the necessary information

● the inquest will enable relatives to hear the witnesses for themselves and, importantly, raise their own relevant questions of witnesses

● the inquest will establish whether steps are necessary to prevent a recurrence of the death

● the inquest will provide some audit of the prosecution policy within the terms of rule 28 of the Coroners Rules 1984, which states:

THE CORONER'S INVESTIGATOR

"If during the course of an inquest evidence is given from which it appears to the coroner that the death of the deceased is likely to be due to an offence within Rule 26(3) and that a person might be charged with such an offence, then the coroner, unless he has previously been notified by the D.P.P that adjournment is unnecessary, shall adjourn the inquest for fourteen days or for such longer period as he may think fit and send to the Director particulars of that evidence."

It should be noted that in most cases the Director of Public Prosecutions (DPP) delegates this function to the local Crown Prosecution Service (CPS).

The government's position paper (2004) states of inquests:

*"We believe that the inquest should remain a **public hearing** (sic) into the circumstances of unnatural deaths, providing an essential safeguard and public scrutiny."* *(op cit paragraph 69)*

The Coroners and Justice Bill Paragraphs 11 – 13 allow for some investigations to be heard by a High Court Judge, with parts being completely private under certain circumstances.

1.08.3 Who is the inquest for?

Some comment that it is a sad state of affairs that inquests are not intended to hold the family in mind. This is an acknowledged flaw - given current society and its expectations. However coronial legislation and raison d'être arose before society evolved to its current state and increased its demands. Consider the dates of Coroners Acts: 1751; 1836; 1887; 1927; 1980; 1988.

Davis et al (2002) in "Experiencing Inquests" state:

"The inquest has travelled so far from its roots. The original intention was to devise a mechanism to examine suspicious deaths." *(Chapter 10 paragraph 67)*

The final report of the Fundamental Review (2003) states of inquests:

"There are widespread criticisms of what is seen as the disparity of practice between coroners in the conduct of inquests and more generally in the way in which they do their work. This is perhaps the most frequent comment that we have heard from families and by organisations such as Railway Safety who work nationally and therefore experience the different handling procedures followed by different coroners." (op cit Chapter 7 paragraph 7)

The government's position paper (2004) stresses:

*"the need to make the system **sensitive to the needs of the bereaved** (sic) and to provide a high standard of service". (op cit paragraph 23)*

1.08.4 Why does a CI attend a scene?
With the reasons for an inquest in mind, the primary purpose of the CI attending is to gather the best possible evidence for the Coroner in relation to these deaths. The best way to gather this is to attend the scene.

The Fundamental Review Report (2003) recognised that the investigation and the inquest are two quite distinct aspects of the Coroner's role (and therefore the CI's role) when it discussed the purposes and scope of death investigations in Chapter 7 paragraphs 36 & 37 and then the choice between an administrative investigation and an inquest:

"A system which continued to have the inquest as the only form of death investigation that is accessible to the family would continue to frustrate many of those involved. There needs to be a general death investigation function which is independent, objective and accessible to families and an inquest system that is designed and resourced to deliver what can be achieved through no other means." (op cit paragraph 38ff)

It benefits:

- The Coroner
- Public – families
- CIs themselves
- Police and other emergency services and other agencies

The presence of the CI throughout the process from scene to body recovery, to the mortuary processes, identification and beyond, ensures accurate and timely information is available to the Coroner. It assists families. It assists the CIs themselves. It can save police resources. These aspects cannot be overstated.

Conversely, absence of the CI may:

- Delay information to the Coroner
- Mean the information may not be complete or accurate
- Hinder families
- Hinder the CIs and makes their working days more difficult
- Cause increased abstraction of police officers from other duties

1.08.5 The benefits of the CI attending the scene

1.08.5.1 Benefits to the Coroner

It has already been acknowledged that the Coroner needs to have a full investigation carried out into any inquestable death. The CI, knowing through experience what a Coroner needs and does not need, may be best placed to carry out that investigation.

The dedicated CI acting on the Coroner's behalf may be able to reduce "out of hours" intrusion on the Coroner. The authority for decision making is vested in the Coroner. The need to telephone the Coroner at all hours of day and night might be lessened with a team of trusted dedicated Investigators. See also section 1.09.5 below.

1.08.5.2 Benefits to families and the public

Society has changed and is constantly changing. "24/7" service is now part of the culture in England and Wales and this applies not only to commerce, but more importantly to service industries.

The public now expect, demand, and perhaps have the right to a "24/7" Coroner's investigative service. The level of this service and the investigation should not vary according to the time of day and the day of the week that a death is discovered. A "time zone lottery" (as opposed to the "postcode lottery") is simply no longer acceptable to society.

The best possible service to the public is a "24/7" seamless service with CIs available to attend any appropriate death, no matter when. This provides the public, families and friends of the deceased with consistency; continuity, one knowledgeable person there from the beginning, at the scene and right through to the final inquest hearing some weeks or months later.

Family members who have not been present at the scene of a death often gain reassurance by talking to a CI who has been there and can answer questions honestly and openly. Accurate contact details can be given to relatives immediately. Continuity is of the utmost importance to a family at a time of grief (anecdotal evidence).

Tissue and organ donation issues can be considered early. This is vital given that time limits are involved. See also section 1.07.2 above.

The Coroner needs to have sufficient evidence for the public inquest hearing itself and the best way of achieving that is to have one person responsible for gathering it all – not an assortment of different people.

If the CI does not attend then who will know what the Coroner wants and needs? The impact on the Coroner will be greater and the Coroner will get more telephone calls from the police at all hours of day and night for decisions.

When a body is legally "under the Coroner's control" it is the Coroner who decides what will happen to the deceased and when and where. No-one else has that legal authority, not even the police. How do the police know what the Coroner wants?

1.08.5.3 Benefits to the CI

With the reasons for an inquest in mind, the primary purpose of the CI attending is to gather the best possible evidence for the Coroner in relation to all inquestable deaths. The best way for the CI to gather this includes attending the scene at the time of the death.

a) It makes the CI's job easier later on if they have attended at the time of the death – and conversely harder if they have not. The CI may have to attend the scene later to take photographs and gather evidence, which is not so effective.

b) The CI gathers information such as the locality; the layout of the building/ area; the inter-personal dynamics between participants. This is the sort of information that does not easily pass on with reports or statements that police have taken, or with photographs. To try and obtain it later is less efficient. Information can be missed which can increase the distress to the grieving family.

1.08.5.4 Benefits to the police

- Releases police officers from scene early, enabling them to carry out other duties which is important as police officers are a valuable resource
- Releases police vehicles from scenes
- Avoids police having to take evidence and property
- Avoids police having to take photographs of scene and of body
- Avoids police having to accompany body to mortuary and deal with property and clothing issues
- Avoids need for Scenes of Crime staff to attend the scene
- Avoids need for police to attend most inquests. CIs have to be there in any case so this avoids duplication of resources. If CIs attend they do their own statements and this avoids need for police to do so

The extent of the role of the CI at the death scene will vary in each police area so not all CIs will do all of the above and in some areas police may choose to retain those tasks.

There will be discussion below of cases where the police will still need to invest many resources (see section 1.12 below).

1.09 Some practicalities for the CI at the scene of a death

1.09.1 Jurisdiction or authority over the body

Whether the police investigate a death or not (see sections 1.12 and 1.15 below), there is a need for the CI to attend the scene. In part this is because the body is legally "under the Coroner's control" from this early stage.

There has been debate over the wording of this unusual relationship between the Coroner and the deceased. "Possession" sometimes causes offence; "control" perhaps less so but still to a degree. In reality however it is the Coroner who decides what will happen to the deceased and when and where. No-one else has that legal authority, not even the police.

In the case of ex parte Kerr (1974) it was stated:

"The coroner's authority over the physical control of the body arises as soon as he decides to hold an inquest and lasts at common law until the inquest is determined."

1.09.2 Information capturing

The CI needs to attend the scene of a relevant death as early as possible, to establish links with the family, friends or witnesses of the deceased and capture their information to be able to take statements from them later. In some cases it may be appropriate to take statements at the time, as long as this suits all concerned.

Certain fundamental information will be needed by the Coroner before he is able to open an inquest, such as the identification of the deceased and the cause of death. The CI can often obtain this information in the initial stages avoiding the need for further questions at a later stage.

If the CI is not involved early, and the police have not invested energy in capturing the information there is a strong chance of evidence being lost. This is not a desirable outcome for the Coroner or their Investigator as there will then be a "cold trail" to pursue at a later time. Not only would this take a lot more time and energy, it may not be successful. The Coroner's full investigation could be compromised.

In police areas where the CI attends, they will often make the arrangements for the post mortem (see section 1.09.6 below).

1.09.3 Body removal

The CI can arrange for the funeral directors to remove the deceased. They will know all local funeral directors, whereas the police may not so well. The CI is likely to appreciate if there is any particular information relevant for the funeral directors. Examples might be:

- An oversize body - so ensure there are more staff attending to deal with the size
- A decomposed body – so bring extra equipment to deal with this
- Multiple bodies - so a vehicle suitable for transporting more than one at a time is necessary
- The body is in a particularly awkward situation – so bring rope, knives etc to gain access

1.09.4 Continuity of identification

Where the CI is in attendance at the scene of a death, they can attend to the continuity of identification. They can remain until the deceased is collected by the funeral directors and then follow the deceased to the relevant mortuary and ensure appropriate labelling. This usually provides a sufficient standard of identification for pathologists and for the Coroner, one of whose duties is to establish the identity of the deceased.

The presence of the CI throughout the process from body recovery, to the mortuary processes, identification and beyond, ensures accurate and timely information is available to the Coroner. It also saves police resources. The CI can make a statement with necessary exhibit evidence included.

1.09.5 Prompt and appropriate evidence gathering

The CI will look for evidence to confirm or otherwise the possible and probable causes of death, and to establish what did or could have occurred, including:

- Examining body for marks and signs as to what occurred
- Questioning witnesses or others to establish circumstances
- Taking photographs and measurements
- Assessing the evidence for its value to the investigation*
- Gathering the evidence they think or know will be needed, at the time, listing it at the time
- Removing the evidence for storage
- Gathering evidence for identification~

*The assessment of the value of the relevant evidence available is a skill that is developed over time. The police do not have the opportunity to work closely with the Coroner in the way that a CI does. Thus they do not regularly gather evidence for a Coroner's inquest investigation and are at a disadvantage in this matter and could potentially miss vital clues. Alternatively to avoid such a possibility the police may retain extraneous material, which can cause logistic problems later for the CI.

There is a potential additional problem with police retaining material which is the potential delay in transferring items to the Coroner's office. Delay enhances grief for family and friends. Delay in returning items such as clothing, mobile telephones, copies of suicide notes or other documentary evidence, is often seen as unacceptable. If it can be avoided it should be.

–The assessment of the value of items in achieving identification is also a skill that is developed over time. The police do not have the need to do this so regularly. This means they may not be aware of the significance of potentially vital clues.

Schedule 4 (3) (1) Coroners and Justice Bill states:

The Senior Coroner, if authorised in writing by the Chief Coroner........ may enter and search any land specified in the authorisation.

So long as certain conditions are satisfied

Schedule 4 (3) (4) states:

"A senior coroner conducting an investigation under this Part who is awfully on any land –
(a) may seize anything that is on the land;
(b) may inspect and take copies of any documents."

Part 1 Chapter 7 allows that the Lord Chancellor may make regulations covering many aspects of coronial law. Paragraph 33 (3) (c) states:

"provision for the delegation by a senior coroner, area coroner or assistant coroner of any of his or her functions, except for functions that involve making judicial decisions or exercising any judicial discretion;"

There is no description as to the extent of delegation. It is expected that some powers will be delegable to CIs, and in particular the powers relating to entry and search and seizure, as part of the investigation.

1.09.6 Post mortem examination arrangements

The CI can make the arrangements for the post mortem including liaising with the pathologist, the most appropriate mortuary and the staff there and sorting out timings. This is especially important when a forensic post mortem is wanted by the Coroner and the police. In other cases the CI will know which is the most appropriate mortuary for any specific body.

By dealing with this aspect immediately the deceased can be moved once, to the most appropriate place, reducing any possibility of delays in the examination. It will also reduce potential distress to the family who often do not like to think of the deceased being "moved around" (anecdotal evidence) if the initial removal is to an inappropriate mortuary. (See also section 1.13.3.1 below.)

1.10 Unnatural deaths not involving suspected offences

1.10.1 Introduction

There is no definition of an "unnatural" death. A specific cause of death may at one point in time be considered unnatural then become natural, such as deaths from the Human Immunodeficiency Virus (HIV) from the early days, now not considered in themselves as unnatural. Deaths from Creutzfeld Jakob Disease (CJD) were at one time unnatural, but no longer (whereas deaths from new variant CJD are still considered unnatural).

Dame Janet Smith commented in The Shipman Inquiry Report (2003):

"It will be observed that I have not sought to draw any distinction between 'natural' and 'unnatural' deaths. This is a distinction that sometimes causes practical difficulty and results in decisions that are difficult to justify logically. The aim of the Coroner Service should be to investigate all deaths to an appropriate degree." (op cit paragraph 19.14)

To further complicate the issue some Coroners currently will want some types of death investigated (therefore invoking the inquest process) that their neighbouring Coroners do not.

The government's position paper (2004) seeks to standardise the deaths that will be referred to the Coroner:

*"Two types of death might be **referred to the coroner**: (sic) those from a list of reportable cases (for example, deaths in custody or deaths following occupational health treatment; see sample list at Annex 2) and, as at present, cases where the treating doctor is unable to certify the cause of death." (op cit paragraph 39)*

In many instances police will attend a death initially for assorted reasons (see below for more on this issue), but once it is established there are no offences the police may not want to invest their scarce resources. However the Coroner still requires a full and thorough investigation.

1.10.2 Examples

Some examples of deaths which fall within this section:

- Deaths which may have initially been treated as potentially involving offences by police, but where they have satisfied themselves they do not need to be involved, e.g. suicides; hangings; drownings; overdoses of prescribed substances; firearms deaths, medical negligence; accidental deaths; fires; poisonings; neglect / self-neglect; abortions etc. (See also sections 1.12 and 1.15 below.) These deaths are often referred to as having been potentially "suspicious"
- Deaths which may require outside expert assistance to deal, e.g. firearms deaths; sub-aqua deaths; deaths involving electricity; Health & Safety deaths. The expertise may also come from police (where the force has a firearms or underwater search unit)
- Deaths in HM Prison establishments. (If not a suspicious death, these cases are not a police responsibility and fall to be investigated by the Coroner. However in many areas the police will continue to be involved)
- Deaths where police have other responsibilities, such as safety or crowd control, e.g. aircraft deaths, paragliders etc; railway deaths. These may be distinguished from multiple deaths / disasters by virtue of the limited number of fatalities and impact (see also section 1.16 below)
- Deaths which may never be reported to the police but are usually reported direct to the Coroner's office, e.g. many hospital deaths, industrial disease; or deaths potentially relating to the deceased's current or past employment

In deaths of this sort the police may not carry out much investigation (on the premise of not investing resources in supporting the Coroner's service unnecessarily).

The government's position paper (2004) states:

*"We see the coroner's officer as having a more clearly defined and consistent **investigative role** (sic) than is often the case at present: going out to take statements from the next of kin or to visit scenes of death, where relevant. In this way, they could take over from the police many responsibilities in relation to non-suspicious deaths." (op cit paragraph 60)*

All deaths in this category will require investigation and will lead to an inquest. The CI should attend the scene for the reasons outlined in sections 1.08 and 1.09 above and should attend before the body is moved at all.

Subsequent chapters will deal in detail with specific types of death that fall within this category of "deaths not involving suspected offences", with guidelines on evidence to look for and specific actions to take.

In deaths such as this the CI will take the lead role, even if the police are present, and will investigate the scene of the death. The police may assist, but they are assisting the Coroner via their Investigator, rather than carrying out enquiries to support a prosecution.

The CI's file will ultimately need to provide evidence to satisfy the Coroner, and thus the public that the death was not a suspicious matter. This may be achieved by the police supplying a report to that effect. In other words that part of the duty can be devolved to the police. Alternatively agreement may be reached that the CI will supply this evidence themselves.

In some instances the police acknowledge the expertise of the CI and look on them as a source of "experienced information" because of their familiarity with death. This is increasingly the case as police recognise that the CIs who regularly attend scenes of death may have a level of knowledge about deaths and scenes that may be greater than the police's own – because of their greater exposure. This may not be appropriate with the obvious violent deaths e.g. the stabbings and shootings at another's hand. However in some cases, e.g. head injuries or hangings, the consultation process is already increasing.

1.11 Apparent suicides

The CI will always want to attend any death that may be as a result of a suicide. This is because such deaths are regarded as unnatural and will need an investigation. The need to hold an inquest in a case of suicide was closely examined in both major reports of 2003. The government's position paper (2004) comments on this issue:

*"We believe that there is real value in holding a judicial inquest. This allows the death to be publicly investigated by a local coroner in a court setting. Two types of death might be **referred to the coroner**: those from a list of reportable cases .... see sample list at Annex 2)." (op cit paragraph 39)*

Annex 2 includes:

"Any violent or traumatic death, including all .... deaths apparently from self-harm."

The CI will always be aware that any apparent suicide should not be assumed to be such - it is possible that it was not. Evidence will need to be gathered to prove suicide and / or disprove other explanations. "Prove everything; assume nothing."

Subsequent chapters will deal in detail with specific types of death that fall within this category of apparent suicides, with guidelines on evidence to look for and specific actions to take.

There is still an offence under the Suicide Act 1961 section 2(1):

"A person who aids, abets, counsels or procures the suicide of another, or an attempt by another, shall be liable on conviction on indictment to imprisonment for a term not exceeding 14 years."

If a person is charged with such an offence the Coroner shall adjourn the holding of the inquest hearing under section 16 Coroners Act 1988 pending a decision as to criminal proceedings. In the Coroners and Justice Bill the adjournment is referred to as "suspension" under Chapter 1 section 14 and Schedule 1 Part 1.

1.12 Deaths involving suspected offences – the police response

1.12.1 Another involved
Where police suspect another person has been involved in a death, they have a duty to investigate to try and detect crime and, if appropriate, secure evidence to obtain a conviction. Such deaths include murder; manslaughter; corporate manslaughter aid and abet suicide and attempts for such offences.

1.12.2 Offences committed
Similarly, where police suspect that offences may have been committed relating to the death but are not necessarily the cause of the death - such as drug related deaths and some child deaths - they have a duty to investigate to try and detect crime and secure evidence to obtain a conviction.

1.12.3 Disasters
Again, where there has been an incident involving multiple fatalities / disasters police will need to consider criminal offences or corporate manslaughter issues and so will want to secure evidence to obtain a conviction. This is as well as their control and command function in such events. (See also section 1.16 below.)

1.12.4 Corporate manslaughter

Increasingly police are considering corporate manslaughter in a number of cases. Some deaths in healthcare settings may initially be referred to the Coroner's Officer (e.g. misadministration of a drug; lack of appropriate treatment). When such a death is shown following post mortem examination to have been as a result of such action or inaction, the CI may refer the death to the police for consideration of systemic issues.

The Corporate Manslaughter and Corporate Homicide Act 2007 has resulted in more referrals of this sort to the police (anecdotal evidence). Section 1 of the Act defines the offence:

(1) An organisation to which this section applies is guilty of an offence if the way in which its activities are managed or organised—
(a) causes a person's death, and
(b) amounts to a gross breach of a relevant duty of care owed by the organisation to the deceased.

1.12.5 Criminal Investigation Department (CID)

In such deaths as those outlined above, police will attend, usually uniform officers as the first response, then CID, the scientific support branch and a Senior Investigating Officer (SIO) who will be a senior detective. The police will consider in many cases appointing a Family Liaison Officer (FLO) to liaise with the family. Further information on police functions and procedures is to be found in the ACPO Murder Investigation Manual (1988 and 2000). See Appendix 1 for designation and explanation of police structure and ranks.

1.12.6 Road traffic deaths

Where there has been a road traffic death the police will usually explore the possibility of prosecution for offences and will investigate accordingly. The ACPO Road Death Investigation Manual 2007 which is available to download from the ACPO website: www.acpo.police.uk encourages traffic police to investigate all incidents as unlawful killings until the contrary is proved. There will be specially trained officers to gather evidence, take photographs and measurements. In each police force the name of the unit to which these officers are attached may vary, e.g. Collision Investigation Unit (CIU) or Forensic Collision Reconstruction and Investigation Unit (FCIRU). The police will usually appoint an SIO and an FLO to liaise with family members and / or other significant people concerned.

It is not necessary to outline the police actions at the scene of such a death here, as these will follow the relevant guidance. The significance for the CI however is that many of the functions they would carry out as discussed in sections 1.8 and 1.9 above will now be performed by the police. For example, the CI would not expect to take photographs, measurements and statements in deaths in this category.

Some deaths are treated initially by the police with a high degree of "suspicion" purely because of the nature of the death, until a very high degree of satisfaction is achieved that the death did not involve another. Then the police will be able to withdraw their resources. Examples of such deaths are: firearms deaths; child deaths; drownings. These are discussed in greater detail in later chapters.

1.13 Deaths involving suspected offences – the coronial response

Where a case is one that the police want to investigate fully (as outlined in section 1.12 above), there is still a role for the CI who should attend the scene for the below reasons (as well as those already discussed).

1.13.1 Coroner's representation at the scene

The Coroner is the person with jurisdiction over the body as outlined in section 1.09 above. Even if police suspect offences and need to investigate a death, the body still falls within the Coroner's jurisdiction.

The Coroner will therefore want representation. Currently this may be provided by the police in some areas, or by the attendance of the CI. In the future it is possible that the police will not provide a support service to the Coroner in the way that many currently do and then a CI will <u>have</u> to attend as well as the police, in order to fulfil this representation.

At what particular stage in such an investigation the CI needs to attend, will vary from case to case and from Coroner to Coroner.

The Coroner knows the police will fulfil their task as regards scenes of crime evidence, photographs etc. Indeed, if there is a suspect, the police will be looking to supply a level of evidence sufficient to secure a conviction at a Crown Court. Such a level of evidence should always satisfy the Coroner if a full inquest hearing subsequently becomes necessary. So a CI may not need to attend a scene early – as part of their usual role is taken by police.

1.13.2 Benefits to the CI in attending these scenes

The early contact with the SIO, Scientific Support Officers and the FLO is invaluable to the CI and thus to the Coroner. The involvement in the continuing process such as briefings provides two way benefits. The CI and the FLO will usually want to visit the family / next of kin together to explain the procedures and anticipated progress of the matter. In such circumstances the CI can reassure the family by their knowledge of the case – or conversely can destroy confidence through ignorance. The family often gain comfort from knowing that the person in front of them was present at the post mortem. The CI can predict the condition of the deceased for viewing after this post mortem process and arrange the timing of it. If viewing is not wanted alternative methods of identification can be discussed.

A case may remain a "suspicious" death if there is a suspect in mind, or in custody, or where it is obvious that an offence has been committed even though there is no suspect at the time. When a suspect is charged the Coroner shall adjourn the inquest under section 16 Coroners Act 1988 pending a decision as to criminal proceedings. In the Coroners and Justice Bill the adjournment is referred to as "suspension" under Chapter 1 section 14 and Schedule 1 Part 1.

Where no suspect is ever apprehended however there will still need to be an inquest. Where this happens, the CI will need to liaise with police to gather the evidence for the Coroner's inquest file. This is not necessarily an exact replica of the police prosecution file. If this happens) the value to the CI of having attended cannot be overstated (see also section 1.15.1 on downgrading below). The reverse is that without it they are almost working blind.

There is additionally a benefit to the CI in attending the forensic post mortem examination (see section 1.13.3.3 below).

1.13.3 Arranging the forensic post mortem examination

1.13.3.1 Who makes the arrangements?

In deaths involving suspected offences, some Coroners "delegate" the authority to arrange the post mortem examination to their local police force, trusting that the SIO will make the most appropriate decision.

The fact that some employers do not pay for their Coroner's Officers / CIs to be on call or available outside office hours may be another factor in the delegation to police forces where this occurs.

However, some Coroners prefer to "delegate" this authority to their CIs, perhaps feeling more secure in their own Investigator, with whom they work all the time, than in a senior police officer who is prone to move from division to division within a force, and even from force to force and therefore from one Coroner's jurisdiction to another.

Another advantage seen with this arrangement is that a CI is more likely to know the relationships between their Coroner and the pathologists available than the senior police officer. Such relationships are built over years of contact in inquests and the post mortem reports supplied and are important. Ultimately, it is for the Coroner to specify which pathologist is to carry out the post mortem examination.

Some Coroners will want a liaison between the police and their Investigator to ensure the best possible investigation – of which the post mortem is an important step. Rarely, however, do Coroners now demand to make the post mortem arrangements themselves - especially at unsocial hours or while in court.

In police areas where the CI attends, they will often make the logistic arrangements for the forensic post mortem, liaising not only with the forensic pathologist but also the most appropriate mortuary and the staff and dealing with the logistics (see section 1.09.6 above).

1.13.3.2 Who has the legal authority?

No matter who physically makes the arrangements, they do so on behalf of the Coroner, - who is the person with the legal power to direct or request a pathologist to carry out a post mortem examination. (See Coroners Rules 1984 Rules 6 and 7 and Coroners Act 1988 sections 19 and 20.)

The police do not have the power to arrange a post mortem examination even in the investigation of crime. The authority is vested only in the Coroner. This is seen by some as a safeguard for society against an abuse as it means that someone independent of the police has the right to choose the pathologist to carry out the examination, and it prevents the police requiring unnecessary examinations.

1.13.3.3 Attendance at the forensic post mortem

In some areas CIs do not attend forensic post mortems. There are a number of reasons why it benefits the CI to attend (see also section 1.09.6 above).

a) It builds up good liaison with the pathologist. The links with pathologists are invaluable and, as in anything, personal contact assists. When it comes to checking on the progress of the post mortem report, or booking the pathologist to attend an inquest (if one is necessary, see section 1.14 below), greater success is likely. It can benefit the pathologist in three main ways:

● The pathologist may ask the CI to take notes. From the pathologist's perspective this is usually preferable to asking a police officer to take notes– on the basis that most CIs at least understand the basic medical terms and the organs of the body and should not need help with the spellings. Although many pathologists prefer to use dictaphones thus obviating any need for note taking, this is not universal

- Where a CI does attend the forensic post mortem they are encouraged to complete a form as per the example at Appendix 2. This can prove invaluable when trying to remember who took the photographs, who was present, who was the SIO, who was the forensic pathologist. It should be a duplicated form, one copy of which is handed to the forensic pathologist, to assist them with their later statement. It can also have additional information added on to it (for example weights of organs) if the particular pathologist finds this helpful. The other copy should remain on the Coroner's file

- Arrangements can be made regarding toxicology and the CI is most likely to know the local arrangements. In many cases the pathologist will send the toxicology through to the Forensic Science Service (FSS), via the police. In some cases, however, double samples are taken with one set going to the FSS (or whoever) and the other going locally. This provides quality control and also a failsafe net. In other cases (see section 1.15.1 below), it may be that the local toxicology is quicker and thus preferable

b) The CI knows immediately how the case is progressing. There is no need to rely on the police to pass the information on in due course.

1.14 Inquests and deaths involving prosecutions

Suspicious or not, in any unnatural death, an inquest shall be opened and adjourned by the Coroner - usually once the cause of death has been established at post mortem and the identification of the deceased confirmed. The CI's role in this opening is to provide the information the Coroner requires (see section 1.09.2 above).

However, a full inquest will not be held if criminal proceedings for a homicide or similar offence (see section 1.12 above) are instigated or if a public enquiry chaired by a judge is established to inquire into the incident. The inquest shall be adjourned under section 16 Coroners Act 1988. In the Coroners and Justice Bill the adjournment is referred to as "suspension" under Chapter 1 section 14 and Schedule 1 Part 1.

1.15 Deaths that "change status"

Deaths may be "downgraded" or "upgraded".

1.15.1 "Downgrading"

There are a number of deaths that the police initially treat as potentially involving offences, sometimes referred to as "suspicious", and thus investigate. The death is subsequently deemed not to require further police investigation or "non-suspicious", i.e. there is insufficient evidence to suggest that offences were involved. It is suggested by some that the number of such cases will increase in an increasingly litigious society.

Police forces prefer to take the attitude that a case can be "downgraded" from "suspicious" to "non-suspicious" if circumstances dictate, far more easily than the reverse.

It would be very costly for police to deal with every case as "suspicious". However, many police forces believe that this is often a cost well spent. Indeed they would rather do this than risk missing evidence by too hasty a decision in the early stages, later discovering that they had needed the evidence after all, when it is too late and the evidence is gone. Each case is assessed at the time. There are few "absolute rules". There are a number of cases where police know at the time that the case is really "non-suspicious", but they think they ought to treat it as such, with a forensic post mortem, "just in case". They are being cautious - to prevent any chance of being later accused of being inefficient. Hence phrases such as "I think it is a non-runner BUT...... just in case". The post mortem is thus a tool confirming their thought processes (or not).

1.15.1.1 Litigation

The increase of litigation being seen in British society generally has an impact on police not wishing to make errors in relation to deaths. It is far easier to justify "over-reaction" than "under-reaction".

1.15.1.2 Consequences of "downgrading"

The consequence for CIs is that many deaths will eventually return to the Coroner's domain, having initially started as a police enquiry. There will then usually need to be an inquest. The CI will continue with the investigation, taking over from where the police leave off. This may be immediately following the post mortem result, in other words the whole investigation is to be done by the CI. Alternatively the police may have taken some statements prior to the point of handing over. (Note that there would not need to be an inquest if following the post mortem the cause of death was found to be natural causes of one variety or another, which does sometimes happen.)

The very fact that "downgrading" does occur, for whatever reason, is further evidence of the advantages for the CI to have attended the scene, as discussed at section 1.08 above.

1.15.2 "Upgrading"

This is when a death starts as a Coroner's inquiry, but later needs police involvement for whatever reason:

- A death that starts as routine may require police involvement after the post mortem examination result has raised concern. In such cases the CI may find themselves in the position of being a witness in police enquiries and in a subsequent court case
- In some cases, a CI may be the initial person to attend the scene of a death, believing it to be one that may result in an inquest and require their attendance. On their attendance the CI will realise that there may be offences requiring police attendance. Early involvement of the police then and there reduces any need for "upgrading" and potential loss of information. Again, the CI may find themselves as a witness in the police enquiries
- A death may initially be attended by police who determine that it is not a matter in which they need invest resources - for example a probable suicide. The CI will proceed with enquiries. Evidence of potential offences may arise during their enquiries. The matter then needs referral back to the

THE CORONER'S INVESTIGATOR

police - along with the information obtained during the course of enquiries thus far. Again, the CI may find themselves as a witness in the police enquiries

- A death is reported to the CI who then needs to involve the police. The need for referral may arise instantly - from the first telephone call received

1.15.3 Transfer of information to or from the Coroner

1.15.3.1 Police to Coroner

In suspicious cases or cases where relevant offences may be prosecutable, the police will take statements to assist them with their prosecution. Such statements are usually made available to the Coroner if necessary at a later date, by local agreement, although there is currently no legal requirement for this to be done. This will assist the CI in not needing to take statements themselves and can reduce distress to witnesses should an inquest subsequently be necessary.

However, in a case where "downgrading" is thought possible or even probable from the start, the police may take very few statements (acting on a basic premise that they will not want to invest time and money in supporting the coronial service unnecessarily). In these cases the minimal amount of police work will be carried out initially – to support or negate any likely suspicion. If the post mortem confirms the police thought processes, that there is no suspicion attached to the death, the case will pass to the Coroner. Any information (relevant to the Coroner's inquest) that has been obtained by the police should be passed to the Coroner's service.

The HOWP Report (2002) recommends the establishment of Service Level Agreements / Standard Operating Procedures (SLAs / SOPs):

"In order to manage the interface between coroners' officers and the police, standard operating procedures (SOPs) (or service level agreements) should be negotiated and agreed in relation to eleven key functions. It was particularly important that SOPs should state where responsibilities lay in all cases." (op cit paragraph 35)

The Shipman Inquiry Report (2003) endorsed the principle of the setting up of these, when talking about the HOWP Report (2002):

"The report recognised the need for adequate provision of transport and equipment and I endorse the relevant recommendations. I also endorse their suggestion that standard operating procedures or service level agreements should be negotiated to manage the interface between coroner's officers and the police." (op cit paragraph 8.51)

SOP6 of the HOWP Report (2002) specifically refers to the engagement of the agencies and the transfer of information.

1.15.3.2 Coroner to police

There are cases where the CI (and / or in future the MEO) begins the enquiry and obtains information, evidence or documentation as part of their enquiries. Subsequently the case becomes one for the police to investigate with offences in mind. In such instances many Coroners will consider favourably the transfer of information to the police. This is again an area which should be covered by an SLA / SOP, as in 1.15.3.1 above

1.15.3.3 Ultimate storage of information

Where documentation, evidence or information is finally stored should be the subject of an SLA / SOP. This should be flexible enough to cater for local wishes as agreed by the Coroner and the police force concerned. In some cases it would seem likely that the police will want to store the originals, letting the Coroner have copies, e.g. in the overtly suspicious cases. At the other end of the spectrum it is likely that the Coroner will store such material where it is clearly a coronial case with no or little police involvement. The most likely area of difficulty may arise where both organisations have been involved.

1.16 Deaths in multiple fatalities or "disasters"

From a coronial perspective a major incident or disaster occurs when the number of deaths in relation to any single incident requires the opening of a temporary mortuary. This may be because the number of fatalities is over and above those that could be dealt with normally and when further resources are required to manage the situation. It might also occur due to the condition and contamination of the bodies rather than the number thereof.

Deaths from multiple fatalities / disasters will be investigated by police as there is always the consideration of criminal offences / corporate manslaughter etc. (see section 1.12.4 above).

Such deaths will usually involve the attendance of CID and scenes of crime department and an SIO and police will often appoint FLOs.

In most of these deaths inquests will be opened and adjourned by the Coroner once the cause of death has been established at post mortem examination and the identification commission is satisfied as to the identity of each particular individual. However, a full inquest per se will quite probably never be held, e.g. should the matter go to Crown Court trial or a public enquiry. In the event that there is a public inquiry the Coroner may hear evidence of identification, medical cause of death, and where the deceased was at the time of his death and where he was found after the incident and leave the "how" to the public inquiry.

The government's position paper (2004) states on this issue:

*"We consider that there should continue to be **certain cases where inquests will be mandatory** (sic). These must include …. multiple deaths after a disaster." (op cit paragraph 70)*

Most of the information about the police response in dealing with this category of death is contained in the ACPO Emergency Procedures Manual (2004). Additionally there will be local major incident plans / contingency plans drawn up in consultation with all relevant bodies, including the local authority, police and the Coroner.

However it is recommended that a CI is present throughout the process from body recovery and through the mortuary processes to ensure accurate and timely information is available to the Coroner. The need to appoint a co-ordinating CI to oversee and maintain an overall view of the situation should also be considered. This is because there will be a need for familiarity with the role of the Coroner and his Investigators in contingency planning, disasters and large-scale deaths.

On the UK resilience website an explanation is given of the role of Coroner's Officers in a mass fatality situation:

"A coroner's officer is the representative of the coroner and duties include supervising procedures for the removal, examination, identification and viewing of victims, and keeping the coroner informed on all matters. The role will be important at the scene of incidents, which they may attend if appropriate, and at the mortuary.
The responsibilities of the coroner's officer include:
- *Providing information for the coroner and contacting hospitals about subsequent deaths*
- *Liaising with victim recovery teams*
- *Arranging transfers of victim from scene to mortuary*
- *Liaising with the lead pathologist on the extent of examination, taking of specimens and determining cause of death*
- *Liaising with local authorities regarding establishment of the mortuary*
- *Membership of the mortuary management team"*
(www.ukresilience.gov.uk/response/recovery_guidance/humanitarian_aspects/fatalities)

The HOWP Report (2002) Annex A section 4 considers the duties of Coroner's Officers in instances of multiple fatalities / disaster.

If the mortuary requirements are more than the local authority can provide, then NEMA is invoked. National Emergency Mortuary Arrangements (NEMA) is a process that is invoked by the Home Office when an approach is made to them and agreed.

A company called KBR, based in Bicester, holds the contract to supply sufficient facilities for up to 600 bodies within 24 – 72 hours anywhere in the country. Additionally, they have the ability to supply extra body storage for up to 96 bodies to supplement local existing facilities, should that be all that is required.

Visit massfatalities.queries@homeoffice.gsi.gov.uk and www.kbr.com for further information.

The UK resilience website contains much useful information including:

"The Mass Fatalities Workstream (under the Civil Contingencies Secretariat Capabilities Programme) aims to build generic capability to deal with large scale events involving large numbers of fatalities both in the UK and overseas.... There is a need to ensure integrity of identification of the deceased whilst balancing the needs of families and any investigation. The ACPO manual is a generic concept of operations for Police Forces and identifies roles and responsibilities. This is currently under review.
Disaster Victim Identification (DVI) Strategy – A DVI manual is in preparation.
Mass Fatality Guidance – Currently under review by the Home office "
(www.ukresilience.gov.uk/response/recovery_guidance/humanitarian_aspects/fatalities)

2

GENERIC REQUIREMENTS AT ALL SCENES

2.01 Introduction

The CI attends the scene of a death or the location of a deceased in inquestable deaths. The role has already been discussed in Chapter 1.

The government's position paper (2004) states:

*"We see the coroner's officer as having a more clearly defined and consistent **investigative role** (sic) than is often the case at present: going out to .... visit scenes of death, where relevant. In this way, they could take over from the police many responsibilities in relation to non-suspicious deaths." (op cit paragraph 60)*

There are certain generic details which can be used to form the basis of a general minimum checklist that can be applied as a template for any death. Not every question on the checklist will always need or be able to be answered immediately. Each individual death will vary. See Appendix 3 for the generic checklist. This has been developed over a few years with the assistance of Coroner's Officers from all around the country, and their collective contribution is acknowledged.

There are also specific headings for checklists that can be applied to particular types of death. These are outlined in subsequent chapters. Sections 2.03 – 2.11 of this chapter consider the headings from the checklist and the rationale behind them.

A generic checklist could be a useful learning tool for a new CI – perhaps attending their first inquestable death without a more experienced CI for guidance. With time the checklist becomes second nature for a CI attending any death. As the CI becomes more experienced the specific checklists will grow. One of the fascinations and challenges of the role of the CI is that each death is different. From one day to the next it is never known what unusual death will occur. The specific checklists may therefore be useful for an experienced CI attending the first of a particular type of death – e.g. a SCUBA diving death.

Specific checklists are to be found in Appendices 10 (falls), 11 (head injury), 12 (Warfarin), 13 (pressure ulcers) and 14 (asbestos related deaths) and a sample investigation plan is to be found at Appendix 9.

2.02 Inquest information requirements

In an inquest case the Coroner registers the death after the full hearing of the inquest has taken place. Thus the CI needs to establish (wherever possible) the full names, date of birth, place of birth, last known address, last occupation of the deceased. Details of the next of kin will need to be ascertained. If the current names are different from the birth names (e.g. by marriage, deed poll etc) documentary evidence may be needed. Issues around gender reassignment need to be approached carefully and sensitively by the CI, but accuracy is paramount.

There are additional requirements for the registration of the death – such as date of birth and occupation of a surviving spouse / civil partner. Not all these details need to be gathered at the beginning of an enquiry. At that point it is information about the deceased's identity that is important. Information about the spouse / civil partner (for example) can wait until later in the discussions with the next of kin.

2.03 The deceased

The Coroner will always need to know details about the deceased. In some cases this may be as specific as the build of the deceased. For example, how did a large person get into a small space? It may be an indication of the force of the water of the fast-flowing stream. That would be a specific.

Background details about the deceased will always need to include any preceding medical condition; whether the person regularly partook of alcohol, drugs or medication; their mental capacity. Where the ME's office has had involvement before a case is passed through to the CI, such information may have been gathered already by the MEO and there will need to be a protocol for passing that over (see 1.02 above). See also the flow chart in the DH programme overview paper 2008 (op cit).

Such basic information can rarely be irrelevant to the Coroner. The Coroner can decide what is relevant while reading the file and / or at the inquest hearing itself. The CI's role is to gather all such information, rather than to filter it out.

2.04 The finder

The Coroner will always need to be told some information about the person finding the deceased, or discovering the incident in which there is a deceased.

Quite apart from the police role in ruling out suspicion, the Coroner also has a duty to negate suspicion when it comes to the inquest hearing. For example, there is a verdict open to the Coroner of "unlawful killing" that does not rely on the police ability to prove a murder, nor on the CPS advice as to chances of successful prosecution. A finder therefore has to be described in relation to any potential involvement in the incident. It is perfectly possible that a "finder" may have been involved in the incident without there being any suspicion cast upon him.

For every finder or person discovering, the best possible evidence for the Coroner will include:
- Who is this person?
- Were they known to the deceased? How long had they known them?
- What was their relationship with the deceased (e.g. colleague, friend, partner, no relationship)?
- Might they have been involved in the incident (to some extent or another)?
- When did they find the deceased or the incident? This to include date and time.
- What were they doing in that location?

2.05 The body

The Coroner will always need to be told about the condition of the body. This is quite apart from any information the pathologist will supply about external and internal examination at the post mortem.

The duty on the Coroner to rule out suspicion applies to this part of the investigation as well. Thus the CI is looking for explanations that account for why a death is not suspicious.

In all cases then the best possible evidence will include:

● Are there any wounds on the body that are not consistent with known former injuries or current incident? This does not necessarily mean suspicion, but might be an indication of a lifestyle – e.g. bruises from regularly falling over while drunk; track marks as evidence of an intravenous (IV) user

● Is the position of the body consistent with the history given? If not why not?

● Was the body moved by the finder for some reason? (not necessarily suspicious). If so when, for what reason and what was the previous position?

2.06 The scene where found

The Coroner will always need information about the scene. Photographs, or even a video, will assist the Coroner enormously and "a picture tells 1000 words". It is much easier for the CI to take photographs to produce to the Coroner as an exhibit than to write a five page statement describing the scene. If photographs fail however – a verbal description is of course adequate and the careful thorough CI will always have notes as a back-up to photographs. In any case photographs do not always tell the entire story.

For example:

● What was the distance between the ligature fixing point and the person found hanging?

● Were the premises secure?

- Are the premises on the ground floor, tenth floor etc?
- Were doors to the property open or closed; locked or unlocked?
- Is there any sign of forced entry?
- Does the CI think this is not suspicious i.e. the person has done this to themselves; or that it "simply happened"? Or might it have been done by someone else and thus require a police investigation?

2.07 Circumstances

The Coroner needs to know as much as possible about the circumstances leading up to the death and "witnesses" will assist with this. In a Coroner's inquiry and inquest a witness is witness as to fact (and indeed hearsay) rather than simply a witness to the death itself. This often needs to be explained to the "witness" who thinks they know little or nothing as they did not see the death.

Circumstances leading up to the death need to be established at least in brief as early as possible to assist the CI in knowing what other questions need to be asked. For example, the fact that the person has previously self-harmed will lead to questions such as:

- How?
- If by self-cutting, on what part of their body did they cut themselves?
- Is that consistent with wounds on the body?
- Have they previously overdosed on medication?
- If so, what medication, how much, was that thought to be deliberated or accidental?

Often such questions need to be answered and brief answers obtained as early as possible before the opportunity to capture it is lost – e.g. a person leaves the area without supplying their details and is then untraceable. As an example, the cliff top rambler who found the rucksack near the edge is a witness. So:

- How did they come to find the rucksack?
- Did they see anyone with it?
- Did they search through it before calling the emergency services?
- Did they remove anything – e.g. to see if the identity could be established?

- Did the wind blow away a piece of paper meaning it is no longer with the property?
- Had they seen what was on that piece of paper before this happened?
- Did they find a mobile phone in the rucksack and use that to call for help as they did not have one of their own?

The answers to questions like this can affect how the enquiry develops from the very start. A full statement does not necessarily need to be taken then and there – this can be done later so long as the contact details are available for the CI. See also chapter 17 on the relevance of notebooks for capturing information.

2.08 The event

If there was a witness to the event itself this information will be vital to the Coroner and such information should be captured. This should happen as early as possible to assist the CI in assessing what other enquiries need to be made and how soon.

For example, if two bodies are found at the foot of cliffs, it is important to know whether ere the two seen to jump hand in hand. This would alter subsequent questions as opposed to knowing that one pushed the other and then jumped himself.

A full statement can be taken at a later time, especially as the witness may well be traumatised. Advice on where to obtain support or counselling will need to be given to such a witness.

2.09 The time

One of the Coroner's primary functions is to establish when the death occurred. Sometimes this may need to be as general as "between x and y". To assist in this process, and if possible to narrow down the time, the CI should look for indications of when there was definitely life – a receipt for example. Also when there was definitely not life – an appointment not attended perhaps, or the first day the milk was not taken in. If a clock or watch or mobile telephone or other mechanical item is referenced for timing, then it is important to check that the time of such a machine is actually accurate, especially around the time of year when clocks go forwards or backwards.

2.10 Actions

The CI needs to keep an open mind in every case they attend, even where circumstances seem obvious. There are dangers of reaching an early conclusion and closing off other avenues of enquiry. A CI should look for evidence to prove or disprove every possible explanation. "Assume nothing, prove everything".

Thus even if a death appears to be from an accident, other theories should be explored and a suicide note should be searched for as thoroughly as possible. Other evidence may be present to indicate planning that goes towards evidence of someone's state of mind. A CI will remember that for the coroner to return a verdict of suicide he has to be sure not only that the person did the act which brought about their death, but that he intended that he would die though that act. Evidence of someone's state of mind will therefore need to be sought in any potential suicide. Subsequent chapters guide the CI to look for and seize all relevant evidence. For example see sections 3.01.4.11, 4.01.2, 4.01.11, 4.04.1.4, 4.05. If death appears to be natural, medications should be searched for and fully detailed to corroborate or disprove the theory.

The safest standard is to seize anything that may be evidence as it can always be returned or disposed of as appropriate at a later date. If the opportunity to seize is lost, it can rarely be revisited successfully. It should not be the case that an embarrassed CI has to give evidence at an inquest hearing that although medication packets were found near to the deceased, details were not recorded of what medication, what strength and how many tablets were missing; nor was the medication seized.

In an age of increasing technology an inquiring mind will need to consider internet usage, mobile phone calls and texts and CCTV as means of establishing evidence.

2.11 Statements

In any inquest case, all things being equal, statements should be obtained from the following where available, as the minimum:

- Next of kin or family members (of which there may be many), covering background information and including identification issues
- The last person to see the deceased alive, or to speak to them or receive an e-mail or text message. Such a statement should include the content of that meeting/conversation etc and the person's demeanour at that time
- Finder, with full details in answer to the section at 2.04 above and any other useful information
- Any other witnesses as to circumstances & background (and this may include friends or acquaintances)
- Any other witnesses covering anything else raised
- Any specialists involved either with body recovery or subsequent enquiries

If police have attended and ruled the death as non-suspicious, the Coroner will need a statement from the senior police officer involved in that process. This should explain to the Coroner why the death was considered possibly suspicious in the first place, – and why it was subsequently ruled not to be suspicious. This is important evidence for the Coroner's inquest where verdicts of "lawful killing" or "unlawful killing" is available and may need to be ruled out.

Additional statements will need to be taken from everyone else who has information bearing on the specifics of each individual death. (See all subsequent chapters relating to specific deaths as well as chapter 13 on statement taking.)

Chapters 3 – 12 deal with specific types of deaths and look at the checklist with those deaths in mind. In each case the generic checklist can be used as a template and the variations added or substituted as appropriate. Thus the generics as discussed in this chapter are not repeated for each deat

3

INQUESTABLE DEATHS INVOLVING WATER

3.01 Drownings

3.01.1 Introduction

In most cases police will consider a drowning to be suspicious until they are satisfied that it is not. A supervisory officer will often attend such a death. The Criminal Investigation Department (CID) may well be called. Once satisfied that the case is not "suspicious" however the police may well reduce their involvement in the investigation. The CI will then need to ask the questions and carry out the investigations prior to an inquest.

As well as the items on the generic checklist, extra things to consider in a death by drowning include:

3.01.2 Wet drowning

The more expected form of drowning occurs when asphyxia leads to relaxation of the airway, which permits the lungs to fill with water. Frothing often occurs around the nose and mouth.

"Drowning consists of filling the lungs with liquid so that oxygen cannot be absorbed. To the extent that this is the direct cause do death, drowning is another form of asphyxia. Further, inhaling water can cause the airway (larynx) to shut or the heart to suddenly stop.... Foam frequently comes from the mouth and nose of a drowning victim, but sometimes this is not visible until pressure is applied to the chest in a resuscitation attempt." (Stone 1999)

3.01.3 Dry-lung drowning

The other form of drowning, more rarely found and not widely known about is dry-lung drowning. Little or no fluid is aspirated. There will be no evidence of frothing.

One explanation is provided in Saukko and Knight (2004):

"The so-called 'dry-lung drowning' is not uncommon, in which the lungs appear normal in all respects, presumably because all the aspirated water has been absorbed through the alveolar walls into the plasma. It has been suggested that this is more likely to occur if cardiac arrest takes place after removal from the water or if laryngeal spasm supervenes to prevent further water entry, so that continued circulatory function is able to clear away intra-alveolar fluid into the plasma." (Saukko and Knight 2004)

Another explanation of "dry drowning" can be found in Stone (1999):

"Since the heart can continue beating for a short time after respiratory reflexes have ended, water absorbed from the lungs unto the bloodstream can be distributed to other parts of the body. Meanwhile little additional water will reach the lungs; hence a dry body with dry lungs." (op cit)

Other explanations include vagal inhibition and reflex closure of the epiglottis.

3.01.4 Specific investigation guidelines – over and above the generic checklist

3.01.4.1 The deceased
- Build of deceased
- Any known medical condition
- Is it unusual to find deceased in this place? Or were they a regular user of the water? E.g. went for a daily swim
- Could the deceased swim? Strong/weak swimmer? Have they had lessons?
- Did the deceased use buoyancy aids? E.g. wings/ring/belt. Were they being worn at the time of recovery?

- Do they have certificates of competency or life saving?
- How often did they swim?
- Had they eaten immediately prior to incident or shortly before? What? How much?
- Had they consumed alcohol immediately prior to incident or shortly before? What? How much?
- Had they taken any drugs (prescribed or illegal) immediately prior to incident or shortly before? What? How much?
- What clothing were they wearing? Shoes? Were they naked? Were they wearing swimming gear? Were they wearing SCUBA gear?
- How long is the deceased believed to have been missing?

3.01.4.2 The finder

- Who is this person?
- Were they known to the deceased?
- Were they intimately involved with the deceased? What is their relationship with the deceased?
- Might the person have been involved in the death and have a part to conceal?
- Date and time they found the deceased

3.01.4.3 The body

- Are there any wounds on the body that are not consistent with known former injuries or current incident?
- Are there any signs that the deceased was forced into the water? E.g. bruises on head, arms (signs of restraint)?
- Is the position of the body consistent with the history given?
- Is there foam from the mouth or nose? Is the foam blood-stained? Was it there when body first recovered – or only when moved?
- Is the hypostasis consistent with the position found?

The importance of a full and accurate description of the state of the deceased when found is vital. CIs need to be aware of this:

"The positive signs of drowning, as opposed to mere immersion, are scanty and not absolutely specific. The most useful ..(is) the presence of frothy fluid in the air

passages – which in fresh bodies, often exudes through the mouth and nostrils. The froth is oedema fluid from the lungs. It is usually white but may be pink or red-tinged." (Saukko and Knight 2004)

3.01.4.4 The scene where entered water (if known)

- What is the point of entry (if can be ascertained)?
- How far is it from where the body was found?
- Was the current going in the appropriate direction?
- Describe the entry point. E.g. river bank/diving board/pier/quayside including height from water at low tide and high tide (if tidal); was there an overhang/a sloping bank/a cliff?
- Have there been other drownings from this entry point? How often? How recent?
- What is the bottom like at this point ? Mud/sand/gravel/boulders/other/unknown
- Is this body of water regularly used for swimming?

3.01.4.5 The scene where found

- How far is it from the point of presumed entry?
- Describe the point where found. E.g. river bank/beach/rocks
- What is the bottom like at this point? E.g. mud/sand/gravel/boulders/other/unknown?
- Is this body of water regularly used for swimming?
- Were there boats on the water? E.g. motor boats/sailing boats/surfboards/windsurfers

3.01.4.6 Circumstances

- Type of water. Pond/lake/stream/river/reservoir/swimming pool/hot tub/jacuzzi/other
- Normal swiftness or rate of current
- Any unusual conditions at the time of the incident
- Weather conditions at time of incident (if known)
- Is it known if there are riptides/undercurrent/shifting sands/whirlpools/underwater holes?
- Are there any known underwater obstructions?

- What is the depth of water (if known)? Note – may vary along suspected route – ensure have as much information as possible
- Is it known how long the deceased was submerged?

3.01.4.7 The event

- Were they seen to enter the water on this occasion? By whom?
- Do we know why they entered the water? Was this recreational? If so were others present?
- Did they fall into the water? If so where from? Boat / dock / bridge?
- Were there freak weather conditions? E.g. flash flood
- Was there a struggle with another or an assault around the time of the incident?
- Was this a rescue attempt? Who was being rescued? Why? Did the deceased remove clothing or shoes before entering?
- Was there an attempt to rescue this deceased? Who by? What happened?
- Was this a SCUBA incident? (see section 3.3. below if so)
- Was this an endurance feat? E.g. a triathlon / channel swim etc

3.01.4.8 The time

- If incident was seen to occur – when did it happen?
- If incident was not seen to occur – what is the state of the body?
- Is there wrinkling of the skin (washer-woman's fingers) that can provide any clue?

3.01.4.9 The rescue/recovery

- Who tried or succeeded in the rescue/recovery? Swimmers/scuba divers?
- What equipment was used? E.g. grapple/rope/lifebelt. Were any injuries possibly caused through this? Describe.

3.01.4.10 In a swimming pool

- Is this a school pool / public / private; other organisation (e.g. scouts); members only
- Were there lifeguards present?
- Was the deceased trespassing – if so what measures were there to keep people out – fences / gates; what condition were these in? Were there gaps in the fence? Were there locks on gates?

- Was rescue equipment kept near the pool? E.g. A ring buoy with an attached line and / or a long handled hook
- Was there a pool cover? Was it in place?
- Were there any buoyancy aids available?
- Were there any diving boards/slides? Were they in safe operating condition?

3.01.4.11 In the bath

- Measure the depth of water in the bath and the depth of the bath itself
- Test the temperature of the water: cold/luke warm / hot?
- Water on the floor/taps still running/plug in plughole or not/bath overflowed?
- Anything contaminating the water? E.g. blood/faeces/urine/other
- Check for other items in the bath. E.g. electric cables or appliances (consider electrocution)/knife/syringe,
- Look for injuries. Turn deceased over then further check for other items in the bath – e.g. knife under the body
- Look for evidence of tablets taken or medication that might indicate natural disease
- Is the deceased clothed/not; face up or face down?
- Are there signs of decomposition? How long the body has been there? Is there evidence of skin slippage or wrinkly skin?
- How warm is the bathroom?
- Is there a gas heater in the bathroom (consider carbon monoxide – see section 4.04 below)
- Was the deceased physically capable of getting into the bath?
- Are there any trip hazards in the room?

3.01.4.12 Other considerations

- Is there any indication of a suicide note? Where? Is it in deceased's handwriting?
- Is there any indication of alcohol or drugs paraphernalia or tablet bottles or packets? Where?
- Is there anything unusual to suggest anything other than a suicide or an accident?

3.01.4.13 Actions

- Take a water sample from entry point and exit point if different
- Look for suicide note(s)
- Take photographs
- Seize any potential evidence

3.01.4.14 Statements

- Next of kin to include background, identification
- Finder
- Royal National Lifeboat Institution (RNLI) (see section 3.02.1 below)
- Coastguard or other official bodies (see section 3.02.2 below)
- Lifeguards (if present)
- Any attempted rescuers
- Any other witnesses as to circumstances, background
- Any other witnesses covering anything raised above

3.01.5 Documentation after inquest

Deaths by drownings are monitored nationally and most Coroners or their Officers will complete a form for ROSPA / RLSS after each drowning. (Royal Society for Prevention of Accidents / Royal Life Saving Society UK). Completion of the form is entirely voluntary and not statutorily required. CIs should ascertain in their individual area whether it is they or their Coroner who submits this form. Either way – the CI should ensure the answers to the questions on the form are established to assist with its accurate completion after the inquest.

3.02 Other related organisations

Depending on where the suspected drowning incident has occurred a number of other agencies may be involved, both at the outset, and during the course of the investigation.

THE CORONER'S INVESTIGATOR'S HANDBOOK

3.02.1 The Royal National Lifeboat Institution (RNLI)

On the front page of the RNLI website www.rnli.org.uk it states:

"The RNLI is the charity that provides a 24-hour lifesaving service around the UK and Republic of Ireland. Our lifeboat service in the UK receives no government funding."

The RNLI may be asked to attend to see if casualties have survived an incident (before it is known whether anyone has died). Indeed, they may be asked to attend to recover a body.

If there is believed to be a body in the water, the local RNLI will be contacted and asked if they will launch. They are not obliged to and will sometimes decline to launch (e.g. if weather conditions are adverse and hazardous).

When the RNLI do recover a body they can provide much information for the Coroner's inquest and the CI should consider taking a statement from the coxswain. This could include information as to the location of the body when recovered (including map grid reference); the condition of the water; how far away from the shore the body was; whether the body was face up or face down; whether there was any other property with the body (if so they will hopefully have recovered that also); when the last low / high tide was. If the body was at foot of cliffs they can advise whether it was above the high water mark or not.

There is a Memorandum of Understanding (MOU) between the RNLI and the Association of Chief Police Officers (ACPO) Diving and Marine Working Group. In the introduction to the final draft of March 2009 it states:

"This document is issued to each chief constable with the recommendation that they should adopt the doctrine and implement it as appropriate in their own force (ACPO Articles of Association)"

3.02.2 Marine and Coastguard Agency (MCA) and Her Majesty's Coastguard (HMCG)

On the search and rescue (SAR) page of the MCA website www.mcga.gov.uk it states:

"The Maritime and Coastguard Agency (MCA) provides a response and co-ordination service for maritime SAR.... The SAR role is undertaken by HM Coastguard, which is responsible for the initiation and co-ordination of civil maritime SAR. This includes the mobilisation, organisation and tasking of adequate resources to respond to persons either in distress at sea, or on those inland waters listed in paragraph 4.2, or to persons at risk of injury or death on the cliffs and shoreline of the UK. As part of its response, HM Coastguard provides Coastguard Rescue Teams for cliff and shoreline search and rescue purposes."

The MOU between RNLI and ACPO (see above) states of the MCA:

"The MCA is responsible throughout the UK for implementing the Government's maritime safety policy. This includes co-ordinating search and rescue at sea through Her Majesty's Coastguard.... Part of the MCA is Her Majesty's Coastguard Service (HMCG)

HM Coastguard

The Government of the United Kingdom assumes responsibility for civilian Search and Rescue (SAR) within the UK and its aviation maritime Search and Rescue Regions.

HM Coastguard is an on-call emergency organisation responsible for the initiation and co-ordination of all civilian maritime SAR within the UK Maritime Search and Rescue Regions. This includes the mobilisation, organisation and tasking of adequate resources to respond to persons either in distress at sea, or to persons at risk of injury or death on the cliffs or shoreline of the United Kingdom." (op cit)

The MCA will respond not only to incidents involving the coast and the sea, but also inland waterways. They have been known to deploy inland (see below). Not only does the MCA have a marine vessel fleet, but also helicopters which are sometimes available to assist police and others. Their personnel (full-time and volunteers) are trained in rope work and often deploy to assist the Coroner to recover a body using these skills.

"Depending on demographics and local risks, teams may be capable of rope rescue (primarily for coastal cliff / steep slope rescue and recovery), mud rescue, coastal search (usually in support of police), preparing SAR helicopter landing sites, meeting vessels which have been the subject of an incident at sea.... However, as in the other emergency services, every task undertaken is underpinned by risk assessment and dynamic risk assessment. Inevitably, Coastguard Rescue Teams (CRTs) are called on from time to time to assist in rescues and relief work inland e.g. quarry rescues, flood relief, missing person searches and in these cases, just as in coastal SAR, the activity is risk assessed with the clear policy mantra that the Coastguard Rescue Service (CRS) will only undertake those tasks for which it is trained and equipped.
The Maritime & Coastguard Agency is committed to a more integrated approach to UK SAR and civil resilience and, bearing in mind that its front-line SAR response capability, the CRS, is made up of volunteers it is, within reason, prepared to respond to emergency situations or assist in multi-agency responses throughout the UK." (Private communication from Coastguard Rescue Service Manager Maritime & Coastguard Agency 2008)

3.03 SCUBA Incidents

SCUBA stands for Self Contained Underwater Breathing Apparatus.

Some additional matters to consider in such a death (as well as those for drowning) and evidence to record for the Coroner are outlined below.

3.03.1 Immediacy of discovery

Many SCUBA diving incidents are reported by others involved in the same SCUBA dive at the time thereof. This section deals with such a scenario. However due to tidal movements etc. a disappearance of a fellow diver may be reported, but a body may not be found for days/weeks/months – if ever. Often the body will be found many miles away from the original diving event, possibly in a different Coroner's jurisdiction and police area. When this occurs there will need to be "cross-border liaison".

As well as the items on the generic checklist, extra things to consider in a SCUBA incident include those mentioned in relation to drownings, above, and additionally:

3.03.2 The deceased

- Were they being instructed? By whom?
- What previous experience did they have of SCUBA diving? Can this be evidenced?
- Is there a personal dive history or logbook?
- What level of SCUBA diving have they previously attained?
- Had they any certificates or evidence of experience in SCUBA diving? What?
- What was the activity prior to the dive? E.g. relaxing/sunbathing/playing volleyball
- Were they wearing full SCUBA gear? Partial?
- Had they consumed any drugs or alcohol prior to diving?

3.03.3 The dive

- Were they under instruction at the time of the incident?
- Was there another diver with the deceased e.g. a buddy? What is their experience?
- How many dives had the deceased done that day? What was the maximum depth of each dive? What was the bottom time of each dive?
- What was the time interval between each dive?
- What time did the last dive begin?
- What was the purpose of the dive? Recreational/salvage/other e.g. to gain certificate for diving (navigation/marine life etc)
- What was the origin of the dive?

3.03.4 The finder

- Who is this person? Was it the buddy or instructor or someone completely different?
- Had they previously SCUBA dived with the deceased?

3.03.5 The body

- Is there anything to indicate whether there has been an incident involving water craft?
- Is there anything to indicate whether there has been an attack by a sea animal? E.g. shark
- Are there signs of drowning? E.g. frothing from nose or mouth

3.03.6 The scene where entered water

- Was this from a boat? Or a beach? Or other?

3.03.7 The scene where found

- How far is it from the point of entry?
- Is it in a direction in keeping with local tides and prevailing water movements?
- Has the weather been different during recent week that might account for difference in expected travel?

3.03.8 The event

- What happened?
- Were any of the recognised distress signals (e.g. low air) given by the deceased?
- Is the first account corroborated by other witnesses or equipment?
- Did the air supply run out?

3.03.9 The rescue / recovery

- If there was a buddy diver did this person make any attempt at recovery?
- What was the rescue attempt?
- Did the rescuers try and share oxygen from their tank?
- If the deceased's air supply appears to have run out – what is the level of the air supply of other divers? E.g. "buddy"
- Did the deceased use a snorkel? If so did they clear the bend of water first?

3.03.10 Equipment

- Note make and type of tank, face mask, etc
- Note any special equipment – such as a dive computer
- Note how many tanks was the deceased carrying / wearing
- Note how much oxygen left in any tank
- Was the equipment their own/rented/borrowed/other? Expand
- Where was the compressed air obtained – dive shop? Portable? On board compressor?
- Who filled it? What others did they fill?

3.03.11 The dive organisation

- Was this a dive school? Is it certified?
- Consider possibilities of negligence/corporate manslaughter and if necessary involve police early on
- How long had the deceased been a student?
- Was it a dive club? How long had deceased been a member?

3.03.12 Actions

- Take photographs of the body with as much equipment in situ as when found as possible (assuming it has not already been removed e.g. in a resuscitation attempt)
- Take photographs of all valves and items of equipment as found including buckles, weight belts etc
- Take photographs of the body as removing equipment – especially head, neck and area where there are injuries
- Seize all SCUBA gear - do not let any dive school take it back to their premises. This includes tank, flippers, face masks, weight belt, regulators, buoyancy control devices, gloves, underwater boards / cameras
- Do not disturb any positions or settings of valves etc.
- If there was a dive computer, seize it and consider calling an expert to interpret its readings
- Seize another tank filled at same time as a comparison
- Consult with Coroner about arranging to have all items tested by an independent tester – consider Health and Safety Executive HSE Diving

Equipment Testing & Examination Service (Personal Protective Equipment Section), Health & Safety Laboratory, Sheffield; or police sub aqua divers; Royal Navy. Note that there may be costs involved in any such tests

- Seize any documentation relating to the deceased's past diving experience
- Request toxicological examination of blood and any other relevant body samples

3.03.13 Statements

- Next of kin – background, identification
- Finder
- MCA; RNLI or other official bodies
- Lifeguards (if present)
- Diving buddy (may be a suspect)
- Diving school proprietors
- Any attempted rescuers
- Anyone who removed any equipment before photographs were taken, describing how items were before they were removed
- Any other witnesses

It is strongly recommended that a Coroner's Office be equipped with a dive manual e.g. the PADI dive manual or similar. If the need arises this should be referred to for useful information.

4

INQUESTABLE DEATHS INVOLVING HANGING & ASPHYXIA

4.01 Hangings

A death by hanging will always require an investigation and if there is no criminal prosecution will lead to an inquest.

4.01.1 Assumptions

The CI should remember that it is very easy to assume that a hanging is a suicide, but it may be accidental or suspicious or auto-erotic. All these possibilities need to be positively ruled out, rather than a suicide being presumed. It is worth noting that most people are unaware of the rapidity of unconsciousness brought about by vagal inhibition and subsequent oxygen starvation to the brain, brought on through the application of a ligature or other similar pressure to the neck.

4.01.2 The deceased

- Is it unusual to find deceased in this place?
- What is deceased wearing? Describe. Is it in disarray or normal position?
- Has deceased put on best clothes? (an indicator of possible suicide)

4.01.3 The body

- Are there any wounds on the body that are not consistent with known former injuries or current incident?
- Are there any signs of restraint: Head injury/restraint bruises on arms/tape marks around mouth?
- Is the position of the body consistent with the history given?
- Is there still a whole ligature or a portion of a ligature on the body?

- Is there a ligature mark on the body? Describe.
- Is the ligature mark on the body consistent with the ligature found at the scene?
- Is there a vanishing point? (see 4.01.13 below for description of this)
- Are there petechial haemorrhages?

4.01.4 The finder

- Is this person friend/family/work colleague/stranger?
- Might the person have been involved in the death and have a part to conceal?

4.01.5 The scene where found

- Indoors / outdoors
- Any signs of struggle or disturbance
- Is there a ligature at the scene (apart from on the body). Does it match the ligature with the body?
- To what is the ligature attached? E.g. door handle/window handle/coat hook/ shower curtain rail/rafter in loft or garage or shed
- Describe the ligature e.g. rope/cloth/wire/cord/flex
- Describe the knot(s)
- Are there other means of suicide? E.g. tablets
- Where is the ladder/stool/other equipment to get into position (if relevant)?

4.01.6 If cut down before CI's arrival

- Who cut them down?
- Were photographs taken first?
- Why were they cut down? E.g. thought possibility of life/wanted to remove from public eye (if in public)/wanted to protect other patients from seeing (if in an institution/hospital)
- Where were they suspended from?
- What position were they in?
- How far off the ground were their feet/knees if kneeling?
- Where was the ladder/stool/other equipment to get into position (if relevant)?

4.01.7 Circumstances

- Describe the degree of planning to achieve the outcome? E.g. how the ligature was set up; how the "drop" was achieved if there was one

4.01.8 The event

- Was the event witnessed? By whom?

4.01.9 The time

- If the event was witnessed - at what time?
- If not, does the body provide any evidence as to the time of the death? E.g. amount of decomposition

4.01.10 Other considerations

- Is there any indication of a suicide note? Where? Is it in deceased's handwriting?
- Is there any indication of alcohol or drugs paraphernalia or tablet bottles or packets? Where?
- Is there anything unusual to suggest anything other than a suicide or an accident?
- Have there been previous suicide attempts and in particular previous hanging attempts by the deceased?

4.01.11 Actions

- Look for evidence to prove or disprove every possible explanation
- Look for suicide note(s)
- Take photographs especially of ligature and knot
- Seize any potential evidence
- If cutting the ligature – avoid the knot
- If cutting the ligature remember to have someone else supporting the deceased's body
- If someone is supporting the body, advise them to wear gloves, not hold the bottom or crutch area, not to have their face close to the deceased's mouth (see section 4.01.14 below for explanation)
- Send portion of ligature to mortuary with body

4.01.12 Statements

- Next of kin to include background, identification
- Finder
- Ensure cover identification of handwriting in any note found in a statement
- Any other witnesses as to circumstances, background
- Any other witnesses covering anything raised above

4.01.13 Vanishing Point

A vanishing point is a point on the neck where the ligature mark is absent. It occurs where the ligature loses contact with the body at the point of strain. It is usually a rising point – consistent with gravity.

Professor Knight describes this as:

"In most instances the point of suspension is indicated by a gap in the skin mark, where the vertical pull of the rope leaves the tilted head to ascend to the knot and thence to the suspension point. This gap is usually seen at one or other side of the neck or at the centre of the back of the neck." (Saukko and Knight 2004)

"Except sometimes when a slip knot is used, the partly circumferential mark will show a defect at the point of suspension, where the vertical tension on the knot carries the ligature away from the skin." (Knight 1998)

4.01.14 Releasing the body

If someone supports a body, they should not hold the bottom or crutch area of the deceased in case of escape of bodily fluids and odours when moved. They should not have their face close to the deceased's mouth as there will be stale air trapped between the ligature point of the trachea and the mouth. The stale air will escape when the deceased is moved – and smells really unpleasant. Apart from not wanting a colleague to experience this – there is always the possibility that they will drop the body if surprised.

4.01.15 Fractured cervical spine

There is a common assumption that hangings will always involve a drop from a considerable height and therefore a fractured cervical spine.

"There are a number of mechanisms by which hanging may cause death, which may act independently or in concert. These include: stretching of the carotid sinus causing reflex cardiac arrest; occlusion of the carotid (and possibly vertebral) arteries; venous occlusion; airway obstruction resulting from pushing the base of the tongue against the roof of the pharynx or from crushing of the larynx or trachea; and finally spinal cord-brainstem disruption." (Saukko and Knight 2004)

4.01.16 The "drop"

Many hangings do not involve a "drop" at all but are nevertheless hangings. Thus a belt from a door handle with the person seated on the ground is quite usual. Similarly the person kneeling and leaning into the ligature. It is important that the CI records all the information available.

4.02 Auto-erotic deaths

4.02.1 Assumptions

The CI should ensure that the evidence does indeed indicate that the death is of this nature rather than a suicide or suspicious death. Suicide can present in a number of ways and may involve some features which could also suggest an auto-erotic death. It will be for the Coroner to determine the verdict – and for the CI to gather the evidence.

4.02.2 Methods

An auto-erotic death usually involves a hanging. However it can also be due to asphyxiation through items placed over the head.

4.02.3 Signs of auto-eroticism

Signs that tend to suggest auto-eroticism include:
- Towel or soft material between the ligature and the neck
- Signs of masturbation

- Mirror located for person to see themselves
- Pornographic material present
- Wearing clothes of opposite sex
- Items of latex or rubber
- Fail safe mechanisms (e.g. knife to cut ligature)
- Absence of a "suicide note"
- Clothing "disturbed" to allow access to genitalia
- Absence of clothing

4.02.4 Investigation guidelines

All investigations and enquiries will be as for hangings or asphyxia as appropriate, with extra photographs of the equipment on the body and other indications found at the location.

4.03 Asphyxiation deaths

4.03.1 Introduction

The Wellcome Trust runs a website in association with amazon.co.uk. The website is: www.forensicmed.co.uk and its front page states:

"Welcome to the only website for medical students dedicated to forensic medicine. This subject is now rarely taught at undergraduate level (particularly in the UK) and so this site provides a unique resource for clinical forensic medicine, legal medicine and forensic pathology."

"Asphyxia ... is usually the term given to deaths due to 'anoxia' or 'hypoxia'.... In its broadest sense it refers to a state in which the body becomes deprived of oxygen while in excess of carbon dioxide (i.e. hypoxia and hypercapnoea). This results in a loss of consciousness and/or death. However, prior to any death the body usually reaches a low oxygen-high carbon dioxide state, and so an 'asphyxial' death is therefore one in which the oxygen deprived state has been achieved unnaturally." (www.forensicmed.co.uk)

Classic signs of asphyxia include:

- Facial congestion, as venous return to the heart is prevented
- Facial oedema
- Cyanosis
- Petechial haemorrhages, often visible in the eyelids, and the whites of the eyes (which may appear quite red), and the inside of the mouth

www.forensicmed.co.uk states:

"The presence of petechial haemorrhages does not automatically point to asphyxia as a cause of death. They are fairly non-specific in that they can be produced whenever there is a marked or sudden increase in vascular congestion of the head that causes rupture of capillaries."

4.03.2 Causes of asphyxia

Other than hangings and auto- deaths, asphyxia deaths can be due to:
- Choking
- Positional asphyxia
- Carbon monoxide – see section 4.04 below
- Other gases – see section 4.05 below
- Smothering
- Strangulation by another

Death by asphyxia does not always give visible eternal signs. It does not even always do so at a post mortem examination.

"There are no specific autopsy findings for 'asphyxia'." (Saukko and Knight 2004)

A death by asphyxia will always require an investigation and if there is no criminal prosecution will lead to an inquest.

4.03.3 Chokings

4.03.3.1 Introduction

Chokings are quite often not reported as such. Indeed they are more likely to be reported as an unexpected death.

This is because chokings are not realised to be such until a post mortem examination which shows inhalation of vomit, gastric contents or pieces of food. In cases such as these the scene will therefore have been removed before the CI is aware that it exists.

Much more emphasis then needs to be placed on witness statements – assuming that there are witnesses to the incident. There often are. Choking on food often takes place in a restaurant and staff may observe. In the elderly they may take place in a nursing or residential care home – and again staff will be invaluable witnesses.

Some hold the view that there are many chokings each year that are not reported at all, because a doctor issues a certificate.

In a choking death it is possible that the CI will not have attended the scene. It is equally likely that no physical evidence will have been recovered. In such a case most of the work for the CI will involve the statement taking.

www.forensicmed.co.uk states:

"When oxygen is not able to reach the lungs because of external occlusion of the mouth and/ or nose, or the airway at the level of the larynx is obstructed (e.g. by a bolus of food), the cause of the asphyxial death is 'obstruction of the airways'. There are no specific autopsy findings that would support the main types of airway obstruction deaths, and circumstantial evidence, physical evidence (e.g. plastic bags used by the deceased) and the scene of death would be relied on to support the diagnosis."

4.03.3.2 Statements for choking cases

In addition to the usual items recorded in statements (see Chapter 13 on statement taking) these will need to cover additionally:

- Was the person self-feeding – or being fed by another?
- Was there any previous history of choking, of food going down the wrong way?
- Is there any known pre-disposing medical condition?
- Was deceased on any drugs that might affect swallowing reflex?
- If self-feeding was there anything prior to the incident? E.g. a noise / action
- If being fed – what happened during the feed? Did the choking occur during the feed or after it had finished?
- What was deceased's position while feeding? Upright, reclining, lying down?

4.03.4 Positional asphyxia

Positional asphyxia will usually involve some reason as to why the deceased could not move to get themselves out of the position that has caused the death. This may be due to intoxication / poisoning (such as alcohol, drugs) that has dulled the person's senses somewhat. It is always advisable to ask for toxicology in these cases.

There may be a physical disease that has led to the problem or a neurological deficit. Illnesses such as epilepsy, myasthaenia gravis or multiple sclerosis and possibly Parkinson's disease could underlie positional asphyxia.

Other causes may include crushing, such as by a heavy weight e.g. a car engine on someone doing mechanics underneath. More rarely crushes can be caused at public events, such as at a football match or a nightclub. Such would be investigated by police, possibly in conjunction with the CI.

"Traumatic asphyxiation is the term given to the condition most often seen after mass disasters, such as the Hillsborough football stadium disaster, or where people have been crushed by collapsing trenches, or by the weight of grain etc in silos. The thorax is transfixed, preventing respiratory movements. There are classic signs

of congestion, cyanosis and petechiae, but there may be no other signs of injury on the body. The florid signs of congestion usually finish at the level of the clavicles." www.forensicmed.co.uk

4.04 Carbon monoxide deaths

"Carbon monoxide's biological effects are mostly due to the fact that it is 200 – 250 times more strongly attached to the oxygen transporting molecule in red blood cells, hemoglobin (sic), than oxygen. A hemoglobin molecule can't carry both carbon monoxide and oxygen. Thus a low concentration of CO in the air can occupy a large fraction of your hemoglobin... Carbon monoxide is also directly toxic to cells by interfering with their ability to use oxygen." (Stone 1999)

In November 2008 the Chief Medical Officer (CMO) issued an update (20/98) on carbon monoxide poisoning. This can be accessed on the Department of Health website and follow the links through cmo: www.dh.gov.uk/cmo. Accompanying his letter there is a leaflet: 'Carbon Monoxide: Are you at risk?' In this leaflet it is explained:

"Carbon monoxide (CO) is a poisonous gas that you can't see, taste or smell. It is released when a carbon-containing fuel – such as gas, oil, coal, coke, petrol or wood – doesn't burn fully because not enough air is available."

4.04.1 Carbon monoxide and vehicles – apparent suicides

As with all apparent suicides, the initial investigation must concern itself with whether there are any suspicions that this is not a suicide – are there things that do not add up? If, after consideration of all the facts, there are no anomalies then the CI can start to consider arranging removal of the body and liaising with next of kin.

If there are anomalies then the police must be involved at the earliest opportunity and afforded all help to deal with a suspicious death that may be a murder / manslaughter.

Carbon monoxide is produced when anything is burned incompletely. Most combustion is somewhat incomplete, so carbon monoxide is produced often. The most common sources of accidental and suicidal deaths by carbon monoxide are vehicles and water heaters, but there are other sources.

Many vehicles emit carbon monoxide. Since 1993 in the UK, passenger cars have been equipped with required catalytic converters. Carbon monoxide is still produced by cars with such converters – it just takes longer to build up enough of the gas to cause death.

4.04.1.1 The vehicle itself
- Make, colour, registration number
- To whom is it registered? Might the deceased be that person?
- Did the person purchase the vehicle with the intention of taking their life this way? Is there a receipt?

4.04.1.2 The location of the vehicle
- Is it close to home? E.g. in garage
- If in garage – was garage door closed shut or easily looked into? Was it locked? Where was the key? Can it be locked from the inside? If not how did the deceased lock it? Is there another access to the garage? E.g. window or loft space
- Is the vehicle in a secreted hidden place – up a farm track, in a wood?
- If so – need to later try & establish how the deceased knew of this location

4.04.1.3 The condition of the vehicle when found
- Was the engine running? Was the key in the ignition?
- If not running was the engine / bonnet warm or cold?
- If not running what position was the key in the ignition?
- Were the doors locked?
- Was there condensation on the inside of the windows?
- Does the inside of the vehicle smell of fuel?
- How much fuel is left in the tank according to the fuel gauge?
- Was the radio / cassette / CD / other audio source playing?

4.04.1.4 The mechanism to convey the exhaust fumes into the vehicle body

- Pipe from exhaust – what sort?
- How is the pipe secured into the exhaust pipe? Tape/material bung/ newspaper wadding?
- What length of pipe is inserted into the exhaust? Is it just lodged in there (indicates a degree of impulsivity) or is there as much as the length of the exhaust pipe will allow (indicates a greater degree of determination)?
- How is the pipe secured into the body of the vehicle? Is there material to fill gap in window etc?
- Where does the pipe go into the body of the vehicle? Rear boot hatch/ rear window?

4.04.1.5 The body

- What position was the deceased in when found?
- Are there any marks on the deceased not consistent with the death or known events prior to the death? If so – consider calling police
- Does the body appear "cherry pink"? (Quite often there are external signs of this phenomenon which is characteristic of carbon monoxide poisoning.) Note that absence of external pinkness is not necessarily a cause for suspicion as the internal pinkness may be quite marked at post mortem
- Had the deceased urinated? (Quite usual)
- Had the deceased vomited? (If so look for tablets as carbon monoxide alone does not usually cause vomiting peri mortem)
- Are there any petechial haemorrhages?
- Is there any relevant history of depression, past suicide attempts or ideations? Past self-harm attempts? Has there been a change in circumstances recently? E.g. marital/physical/financial/emotional status

"The classical 'cherry-pink' colour of carboxyhaemoglobin is usually evident if the saturation of the blood exceeds about 30 per cent... below 20 per cent no coloration is visible." (Saukko and Knight 2004)

4.04.1.6 The finder

- Who found this?
- What were they doing to find it/why were they there?
- What action did they take? E.g. try all doors/smash window/pull pipe mechanism out of exhaust pipe or out of car body

4.04.1.7 The interior of the car – evidence

- Is there a "suicide note"? Where was it found?
- Is there a receipt for fuel? How recent? (often people will go and fill up specifically for the purpose)
- Is there evidence of tablets? If so list amounts, details etc. (Often people will take tablets as well as a failsafe mechanism)
- Are there empty food and drink containers? If so list and details of location (people often eat sweets/chocolate/crisps and/or drink alcohol/soft drinks with an attitude of "might as well die happy")
- If there was music playing – what radio channel, CD or cassette? (people often choose their favourite or something of special significance)
- Is there paraphernalia to do with the mechanism?
- Are there scissors or knife to cut the hosepipe? If so is there packaging for it? (often people will buy a brand new pipe from a store for the purpose)
- Is there more hosepipe? (often people will buy a brand new pipe from a store for the purpose) If so – do the cut ends appear to match?
- Is there more tape? (often people will buy a brand new reel of tape from a store for the purpose) If so – do the cut ends appear to match?
- Are there spare rags/newspapers etc to fill the gaps?
- Are there receipts for any of these items? (often bought immediately prior and receipt and credit card dockets still in car or person's wallet)

4.04.2 Carbon monoxide and places of residence

4.04.2.1 Manslaughter

As with all deaths, the initial investigation must concern itself with whether there are any suspicions that a crime may be involved. If there are any concerns then the police must be involved at the earliest opportunity so they can consider a suspicious death that may be a murder / manslaughter. They may consider issues of corporate manslaughter under the Corporate Manslaughter and Corporate Homicide Act 2007.

In cases such as this there is also the possibility of a corporate manslaughter under certain conditions. More likely, however is that the Health and Safety Executive will want to investigate to see if offences have been committed – e.g. by landlords.

In the CMO 2008 leaflet Carbon Monoxide: Are you at risk? as mentioned above it states:

"landlords have a legal duty to have any gas appliances they provide, including cabinet heaters and flues, checked annually and to provide ... with a copy of the safety check record. Landlords also have a legal duty of care." (op cit)

4.04.2.2 Accidents

As with all apparent accidents, the initial investigation must concern itself with whether there are any suspicions that this is not an accident – are there things that do not add up? If after consideration of all the facts, there are no anomalies then the CI can start to consider removing the body and dealing with next of kin.

In the CMO 2008 leaflet Carbon Monoxide: Are you at risk? It states that carbon monoxide can be released:

".. when appliances such as room and water heaters, fires and cookers have been wrongly Installed or poorly maintained, or when a chimney, flue or air vent into the room such as an air brick has been fully or partially blocked. Poor ventilation adds to the problem by allowing CO concentrations to build up. Anyone spending time with faulty appliances will be affected. Accidental exposure to CO kills more than 50 people each year in England and Wales. It can kill without warning, sometimes in a matter of minutes." (op cit)

4.04.2.3 Scene

- Obtain a description of the scene, including the temperature. If it is hot – the heat source may still be on but not burning fully; if cold the heat source may have extinguished (e.g. a pilot light) but the gas source still being supplied
- Consider your own safety first of all
- Is there a possible source of carbon monoxide?
- Is there a paraffin heater, gas appliance?
- Is there a vent for the appliance? Is it blocked or obviously defective (even without an engineer)?
- Is the appliance being used in a non-vented area?
- Was a gas oven being used as a source of heating?
- Was a camping gas stove being used (e.g. in a tent)
- Is there an integral garage – if so could the source be from the garage?
- Are there other deceased people or even animals?

4.04.2.4 Buildings

- Does the deceased own the property?
- Is it rented? Who is the landlord? Are there other cases of similar in properties owned by the same landlord? (Consider HSE)
- Is there any evidence of a service history for the suspected appliance?

4.04.2.5 Mobile homes, camper vans, caravans

- Make, colour, registration number / serial number
- To whom is it registered? Might the deceased be that person?
- Is there an appliance inside that was the cause or is it the vehicle's heater?

4.04.2.6 Boats

- Was the deceased tailboarding on the back of the boat where the exhaust comes out? Have they done this before?

4.04.2.7 Actions

- Seize any evidential items

4.04.2.8 Documentation after inquest

Deaths involving accidental deaths from carbon monoxide poisoning are monitored nationally and most Coroners or their Investigators will complete a form for the Carbon Monoxide and Gas Safety Society after each such case. Completion of the form is entirely voluntary and not statutorily required. CIs should ascertain in their individual area whether it is they or their Coroner who submits this form. Either way – the CI should ensure the answers to the questions on the form are established to assist with its accurate completion after the inquest.

4.05 Other gases

Helium, argon, nitrogen, neon and butane can all cause death. Helium is now becoming less unusual (anecdotal) perhaps because of the availability of helium for balloon kits. Such kits are available on the internet and local toy stores and not expensive. Helium is an inert gas that "flushes" oxygen out of the body.

The deliberate choice of a death by such means usually involves a plastic bag being affixed over the head. The bag could be one from a supermarket, although these tend to have holes in the bottom which can prove a disadvantage when used for this purpose. It is now possible to buy a specially designed, pre-manufactured bag which has plastic tubing feeding into it through a sealed flange that is leak-proof. The bag even comes with elastication to secure it in place around the neck. Equipment such as helium canisters and pre-manufactured bags may be taken by the Coroner as evidence of intent. An accompanying dosage of alcohol or medication is not unusual and so should be looked for. It is not unusual to find literature from organisations such as Dignitas, or Friends at the End and even books and DVDs such as "Final Exit" which provide details and even video demonstrations.

Dignitas is one 'right-to-die' organisation in Switzerland that has attracted much media interest in recent years.

Friends at the End is a members' democratic society, dedicated to promoting knowledge about end-of-life choices & dignified death. It supplies a quarterly newsletter to its members. Visit their website: www.friends-at-the-end.org.uk for more information which may assist the Coroner.

The CI's actions will be the same at the scene of such a death as for any other possible suicide and the generic checklist (see Chapter 2) as well as points raised in earlier sections in this chapter will prove useful.

4.06 Smothering

The Compact Oxford Dictionary defines "smother" as:

"suffocate by covering the nose and mouth"

The term "smothering" usually implies that another has had a hand in the process, although strictly that is not part of the above definition. Of course, if another is suspected of being involved then the police will treat the death as a "suspicious death". See Chapter 1 for more discussion on the process in such circumstances.

4.07 Strangulation by another

Again, if another is suspected of being involved then the police will treat the death as a "suspicious death". See Chapter 1 for more discussion on the process in such circumstances.

5

INQUESTABLE DEATHS INVOLVING OTHER AGENCIES

5.01 Introduction

5.01.1 Benefits and disadvantages

The involvement of other agencies can be of both benefit and disbenefit to the Coroner's inquest process.

Each agency exists for its own reason, however laid down. It is not there to provide an impartial independent inquisitorial approach to an investigation of any death.

This was recognised in the report of the Fundamental Review Report (2003):

"... statutory air accident, maritime and railway investigations. Their purpose is to find out what caused the incident and make recommendations for technical systems change which would make it less likely to happen again." (op cit Chapter 10 paragraphs 12 and 13)

The police have many duties including preservation of life and property but in relation to Coroners' cases they may ask themselves "Is there any prosecution to be brought in this matter?" Similarly for the HSE (see section 5.08 below).

It may be suggested that there is a disadvantage in that another agency is taking evidence for a specific and perhaps narrower purpose than the Coroner's interest. This is usually looking towards a prosecution that is, of course, no concern of the Coroner.

In pursuing their enquiry another agency may miss issues that the Coroner is concerned with. They may only take the narrow view – not look at the wider whole. Thus gaps can occur and supplementary statements may have to be taken by the CI.

The Coroner has to balance the use of enquiries and their results by such other agencies against the potential "lack of independence". In using information obtained by any other agency the duplication of provision of information is avoided. This of course is helpful to the information provider, in that no-one likes to have to repeat information to two or more different agencies.

The Fundamental Review Report (2003) states:

"We suggest that:
a. the inquest, or a coroner's investigation, would be the main official process for identifying the circumstances of death of individuals;
b. where a technical investigation had been conducted by statutory body such as the Air Accident Investigation Board its technical inquiries and investigations should not be unnecessarily repeated or duplicated by the inquest or the coroners' (sic) investigators." (op cit Chapter 10 paragraph 52)

Even where there is another agency producing a report and the Coroner indicates that this is likely to be satisfactory, the CI should remain proactive. Quite apart from the family care, the necessity to liaise effectively with the specialists cannot be over-emphasised.

Strategies should be agreed covering:
● Who is going to do what?
● Who will liaise with the media/press?
● Who will tell next of kin what information at what stage? (This is to avoid confusion, and not to withhold information from those who have the right to know it)

The CI needs to regularly check on progress of the report with the specialist – otherwise there is a possibility of delays. The family and the Coroner need updating about the progress at regular intervals.

There are specific instances when a Coroner's enquiry needs to be seen to be completely independent of any other agency. This applies specifically to investigations carried out by the prison service or by the police - particularly into deaths in police custody (see also Chapter 6 on this issue). It also applies to deaths within an NHS Trust – see Chapter 11 on Deaths in Secondary Healthcare Settings.

The government's position paper (2004) comments:

*"special arrangements will be needed where **other investigations** (sic) about the death or circumstances of the death are also underway (for example, criminal proceedings). In general the coroner's work would, as now, wait upon their outcome. We do not think that a coroner (sic) should be obliged to investigate a death, when he or she is satisfied that it has already been adequately investigated by other means." (op cit paragraph 71)*

5.01.2 Specialist CIs

There is a case for specialist CIs who should deal with certain categories of death. This was considered by both the recent major reviews.

The Fundamental Review Report (2003) suggests:

"Each area coroner's office would employ on average around 10 Coroners' Officers to handle the casework, liaison with families, and do some investigations. They would have a mixture of investigative and healthcare skills. In each office there would be some specialisation, for example in child deaths, self-inflicted deaths and workplace deaths." (op cit Chapter 15 paragraph 93)

The Shipman Inquiry Report (2003) comments on specialisation of skills for CIs also:

"I envisage that some investigators.... would develop skills for the investigation of the circumstances of deaths, for example deaths in the workplace." *(op cit 19.20)*

5.02 Road Traffic Deaths

5.02.1 The investigation

The police will usually carry out the investigation into these deaths and such an investigation is usually acceptable to the Coroner. The obvious concern would be when the collision / incident involved a police officer or police vehicle. Such cases however are usually overseen by the Independent Police Complaints Commission (IPCC) to provide a degree of independence. The IPCC took over from the Police Complaints Authority on 1st April 2004. Their enquiries may satisfy the Coroner's requirement for an independent investigation.

Even in a fatal RTC case there may be enquiries that the Coroner will be concerned with, that the police do not make. For example, evidence of a deceased's previous relevant medical history; information about deafness; poor eyesight - these may not be of great importance to the police prosecution process. However they will be of interest to the Coroner and the CI may take additional statements e.g. from a general practitioner.

The government's position paper (2004) includes "all traffic deaths" in the list in Annex 2 of those still normally requiring a judicial inquest.

The Senior Investigating Officer (SIO) will usually be a trained Traffic Division supervisor. The SIO is responsible for setting policies, lines of enquiry, actions and direction for the police investigation.

5.02.2 The aims of the CI at this sort of death are to:

- Ensure the Coroner receives the highest possible level of evidence available in every case
- Ensure effective links are established with the police investigative team from
- Liaise with family at an early stage

5.02.3 The primary role of the CI in an RTC death is to:

- Attend the scene
- Deal with identification issues
- Establish and maintain links with the family, the SIO, the FLO and the FCIRU officer
- Facilitate the smooth progress of the case to the Coroner's inquest

As well as the items on the generic checklist, extra things to consider include:

5.02.4 The deceased

- Is it usual for the deceased to be in this location?
- Is it usual for the deceased to be in this vehicle?
- Be they a passenger, a driver or a pedestrian, the issue of alcohol is of particular import in a road traffic collision death. How much might this have impacted on the final outcome?
- Similarly as regards drugs, prescribed or otherwise

5.02.5 The person reporting the Road Traffic Collision (RTC)

- What vehicle was this person in (if any)?

5.02.6 The body

- Is there anything unusual that might have a bearing on the case?
- Is there evidence to support or disprove seatbelt usage?
- Did the airbag(s) activate?

5.02.7 The event

- Was the event witnessed by anybody independent of the collision itself?

5.02.8 Actions at the scene

- Deal with identification issues
- Establish and maintain links with any family / friends present
- Liaise with the SIO
- Liaise with the FLO if known at this stage – either in person if at scene or by telephone if not. Ensure aware of any family liaison strategy arranged at this early stage
- Liaise with the FCIRU officer
- Arrange funeral directors' attendance, then follow body(ies) to mortuary. This deals with continuity of identification issues
- Establish likelihood of prosecution for section 1 or section 3A Road Traffic Act RTA 1988 (as amended by s1, s3 RTA 1991) or; S2B, s3ZB RTA 1988 (as amended by s20, s21 Road Safety Act 2006) offences
- Ascertain what needs police have from immediate actions – e.g. seizure of clothing/property at mortuary

5.02.9 Actions away from the scene

5.02.9.1 At mortuary

- Undress body(ies)
- Preserve clothing - for police investigations if an issue, or for families to choose if they want them back later
- Preserve property - establish if any relevant for police enquiries, if not be able to hand back to family, fully documented
- Assess suitability for tissue donation
- Assess state for viewing/identification so can better inform family

5.02.9.2 Away from mortuary

- Maintain log for the duration of the case to inquest conclusion (this log could be disclosable in any subsequent prosecution)
- Document all contact or attempted contact with officers or family in the Coroner's Inquest Log
- Be aware of the force traffic policy contact assessment levels regarding each contact with the family & adopt the same assessment levels for each case

- Maintain contact with the relevant FLO(s) to liaise over issues such as property, identification, tissue donation and other procedural matters if not already resolved
- Facilitate contact between the family and support agencies as appropriate (bearing in mind that the FLO also does this)
- Establish likelihood of prosecution for section 1 or section 3A RTA 1988 (as amended by s1, s3 RTA 1991) or S2B, s3ZB RTA 1988 (as amended by s20, s21 Road Safety Act 2006) offences if not already established at the scene
- Contact National Blood Service Tissue Services if appropriate in accordance with family's wishes for tissue donation consideration

5.02.10 Statements

- From relevant people – may be more than one and they may not agree with each other. Should also deal with health, mobility, hearing and eyesight issues relating to deceased – if not covered by police

The relevance of the specific road traffic offences mentioned above relates to the fact that if a person is charged with any such offence the Coroner must adjourn an inquest under section 16(1)(b) Coroners Act 1988. This therefore means that, just as for a person charged with murder or manslaughter, there is the right to ask the Coroner for a second post mortem examination. See Matthews (2002) for further information on this as it applies to 'properly interested persons'. The CI always needs to be aware of such situations so as not to give the family the wrong information about how soon the deceased's body will be released. Hence the need to establish as early as possible whether such offences are being considered by the police following a road traffic collision

5.02.11 Road deaths and the Health and Safety Executive (HSE)

Sometimes a road traffic death will also involve the HSE as a death in the workplace. There is an Operational Minute from 2003 available to download from the HSE website which provides the HSE policy.

"on enforcement of health and safety legislation in relation to work-related road traffic incidents. It gives guidance on the type of work-related road traffic incidents where inspectors are likely to have a regulatory role. It deals primarily with demarcation of enforcement responsibility." (Work-related road traffic incidents: an explanation of circumstances where HSE may have a role to play (2003))

5.02.12 Documentation after inquest

Deaths involving road traffic collisions are monitored nationally and most Coroners or their Investigators will complete a form for the Transport Research Laboratory. Completion of the form is entirely voluntary and not statutorily required. CIs should ascertain in their individual area whether it is they or their Coroner who submits this form. Either way the CI should ensure the answers to the questions on the form are established to assist with its accurate completion after the inquest.

5.03 Aircraft deaths

The Air Accident Investigation Board (AAIB) investigates all aircraft crashes.

"The UK Air Accidents Investigation Branch (AAIB) is part of the Department for Transport and is responsible for the investigation of civil aircraft accidents and serious incidents within the UK." www.aaib.dft.gov.uk

They produce an in-depth report which is usually acceptable to a Coroner for their inquest. This should avoid the issue of duplication (see section 5.01 above). It will cover all the relevant information as discussed below. Certain aspects are highlighted here to raise awareness of the sort of information the AAIB produces. The importance for the CI is to gather the information for the Coroner as early as possible and to liaise over the immediate practicalities concerning identification, post mortems and inquest opening procedures.

The AAIB have produced some leaflets which are available to download from their website www.aaib.dft.gov.uk including:

The Investigation of Accidents or Serious Incidents to Public Transport Aircraft; and The Investigation of Accidents to General Aviation Aircraft

Everything about aircraft deaths depends on the size of the incident, from a jumbo jet to a single seater plane; from a commercial situation to a pleasure flight.

The government's position paper (2004) includes "any violent or traumatic death" in the list in Annex 2 of those still normally requiring a judicial inquest. It is difficult to envisage how an aircraft death would fall outside this categorisation.

5.03.1 The deceased

Ensure the identity is accurate – especially at an air show where the name the organisers have may be different to the actual pilot/occupant.

Identification may be a particular problem in cases such as this (see Chapter 14 for more on identification).

5.03.2 Circumstances

Obviously the circumstances will be vital to the Coroner. Some questions will include:

● Was the incident an air show?
● Was it a private or commercial aircraft?
● Where did it start its flight?
● Was it under hire or privately owned? Being flown commercially or for pleasure?
● Who has died – pilot, crew or passenger?

There are many more questions all dependent on the type of aircraft and circumstances. All should be answered by the AAIB report.

5.03.3 The event

If this was at an air show it is probable that there are a large number of witnesses and the danger is of too many offers of information rather than the more usual case of too few witnesses. The immediate broadcasting by the media will create problems of an unusual nature for a CI. Relatives may know about the crash before it is known who the relatives are. Air traffic control should be able to provide information about what actually happened in a "non show" situation.

5.03.4 Actions at the scene

- Start thinking of dealing with identification issues
- Liaise with the SIO
- Liaise with the FLO(s) if known at this stage – either in person if at scene or by telephone if not. Ensure aware of any family liaison strategy arranged at this early stage
- Establish contact with AAIB representative at an early stage
- Be mindful of additional health and safety hazards e.g. aviation fuel
- Arrange funeral directors' attendance. Then follow body(ies) to mortuary, dealing with continuity of identification issues

5.03.5 Actions away from the scene

5.03.5.1 At mortuary

- Preserve body in state recovered for special pathologist
- Attend post mortem on behalf of Coroner

5.03.5.2 Away from mortuary

- Maintain log for the duration of the case to inquest conclusion (this log could be disclosable in any subsequent prosecution)
- Facilitate contact between the family and support agencies as appropriate (bearing in mind that the FLO also does this if appointed)
- Ensure details of pilot's licences are obtained (eg private pilot's licence/ commercial pilot's licence/air transport pilot's licence). Was the licence appropriate?

- Establish any licence requirements. Have they been complied with?
- Establish how many flying hours the pilot has
- Ensure details of maintenance of the aircraft are obtained
- Establish whether the maintenance company has itself been appropriately certified

5.04 Railway deaths

5.04.1 Introduction

The Rail Accident investigation Board (RAIB) investigates all major disasters or multiple fatalities.

"The Rail Accident Investigation Branch (RAIB) is the independent railway accident investigation organisation for the UK. It investigates railway accidents and incidents on the UK's railways." www.raib.gov.uk

The role of the CI at such an occurrence is briefly considered in Chapter 1 and is mainly liaison.

There is a Memorandum of Understanding agreed between the Rail Accident Investigation Branch, the British Transport Police, Association of Chief Police Officers and the Office of Rail Regulation for the Investigation of Rail Accidents and Incidents in England and Wales (2006). This sets out the roles and responsibilities of the organisations, and the interface between them. It can be downloaded from the RAIB website: www.raib.gov.uk.

There is a Memorandum of Understanding between the Coroners' Society of England and Wales and the Office of Rail Regulation signed on 26th August 2008 and available to download from the ORR website www.rail-reg.gov.uk.

"It is intended to promote and continue effective working relationships between Coroners and HM Inspectors of Railways, with the object of fostering constructive cooperation." www.rail-reg.gov.uk

Single fatalities on railways are not unusual and the CI can expect to deal with such cases regularly. In some areas the British Transport Police Force (BTPF, but more usually known as BTP) produces a report which is usually acceptable to a Coroner for their inquest. The issue of duplication could then be avoided (see section 5.01 above). It should cover all the relevant information as discussed below. However in other areas the investigation is left to the CI.

If BTP are assisting, the importance for the CI is to gather the information for the Coroner as early as possible and to liaise over the immediate practicalities concerning identification, post mortems and inquest opening procedures. If CIs are to carry out their own investigation more work will be required. In this section it is assumed that the CI will do the investigations. Accordingly as well as the generic checklist the below are important:

5.04.2 The deceased

- How long is the deceased believed to have been missing?
- Any previous self-harm or suicide attempts known?
- Any previous visits to the location? (possibly practice runs)

5.04.3 The body

- Describe clothing (may be important in CCTV investigations; may be relevant as regards visibility issues)
- Is the position of the body consistent with the account given?

5.04.4 The scene where found

- Is this at (or close to) a railway station?
- If not – how is access to this part of the railway gained? – was person seen gaining access to railway line?
- Is there electrification at this point?
- How many rail lines are there?

5.04.5 The event

- Was the event witnessed?
- How long had deceased been in position prior to incident?

- Was this the first train (and first opportunity) since deceased had been in position or had other trains gone past in the interim? If so – is it known why they chose this train?

5.04.6 Actions

- Measure distance from presumed access point(s) to where body believed to have been struck
- Look for other belongings up and down the track
- Obtain sketch plan of scene – including measurements of width between rails, gaps between sets of tracks; height between top of trains and bottom of bridge (if bridge involved); height between top of trains and bottom of gantry or other object in collision with
- Obtain CCTV of station where occurred showing movements and actions and demeanour of deceased – and movement of others (to establish lack of suspicion)
- If incident occurred other than at a station – check CCTV of stations up and down track to see where access gained, what time, manner of deceased on the CCTV, was anyone else with the deceased?
- Liaise with RAIB – if appropriate
- Liaise with BTP (who liaise with ORR)

5.04.7 Statements

- Identification – consider how this could or should be done
- Train driver; train conductor
- Other passengers on train (including negative evidence). To include movements and actions of deceased prior to incident – e.g. seen to go to door and open it/seen to put head out of window/seen to climb on to roof
- Other passengers at station – describing movements and actions of deceased prior to incident – e.g. seen to walk on to track/seen to jump into path of oncoming train

5.04.8 Documentation after inquest

There are a myriad of different forms that the Coroner completes after inquests into various categories of death. Most of these forms are voluntary and some Coroners regard this as a part of their social function – of better informing the interested bodies of the findings of an inquest. Thus in a drowning case (see section 3.01 above) a form is completed for RoSPA; in a death involving horses a form is completed for the British Horse Society etc.

However the only statutory requirement for the Coroner to supply information such as this, is in relation to railway fatalities.

Section 11(8) Coroners Act 1988 states:

"In the case of an inquest into the death of a person who is proved:-
(a) to have been killed on a railway; or
(b) to have died in consequence of injuries received on a railway,
the Coroner shall within seven days after holding the inquest, make a return of the death, including the cause of death, to the Secretary of State in such form as he may require; and in this subsection "railway" has the same meaning as in the Railway Regulation Act 1842."

The CI should ensure that the information the Coroner will need to complete the form is obtained to assist with its accurate completion after the inquest.

CIs may also be aware that in 2004 the British Transport Police Authority (BTPA) came into existence under the provisions of the Railways and Transport Safety Act 2003. The BTPA assumed the role and responsibilities of the Strategic Rail Authority (SRA) as employer of the BTP.

5.04.9 Statutory referral of certain deaths to relevant authority

This aspect of voluntary or statutory reporting after an inquest is quite distinct from the obligation to inform various bodies of an occurrence involving a death as early as possible after that death has occurred. This includes deaths requiring referral to the Health and Safety Executive (HSE), Air Accident

Investigation Board (AAIB), Marine Accident Investigation Board (MAIB) and Rail Accident investigation Board (RAIB).

5.05 Deaths involving fires

5.05.1 Introduction

Initially the local fire service will be in attendance at any fire involving a fatality. A Senior Fire officer or expert from the local fire service will make an initial assessment as to whether the scene is suspicious or not. Usually a fire expert from the Forensic Science Service (FSS) will be called in by police if thought appropriate through concern of either the police or local fire service.

The fire experts will carry out their own investigation to look at the cause of the fire and its spread and progress.

If the matter is thought to be suspicious or probably suspicious, the police will appoint an SIO to work alongside the fire service SIO and If it is thought to be so the Police Scientific Support Branch will attend in the usual way.

The role of the CI at the scene of a death by fire is therefore largely affected by whether it is considered suspicious or involving arson or not.

The CI does not need to enter the scene in cases such as these – for the same reason as for any other suspicious death.

If it is thought not to be suspicious there is no reason why the CI should not enter the scene – apart from any health and safety requirements as advised by the fire service. Indeed it may be helpful in subsequent dealings with the family who may not feel able to enter the scene at any stage but nevertheless want to know some information. If the family do subsequently want to enter the scene after it has been made safe by the Fire Service. It may fall to the extended role of the CI to support the family. In these cases knowledge of the facts may assist the family.

5.05.2 The deceased

- The issue of alcohol and drugs may be of particular import in cases involving fires
- Did someone from the premises have the habit of leaving a lighted oven, or a lighted gas or electric ring on to provide heat to the house?
- The issue of smoking will be of particular importance
- What was the previous physical status of the deceased? E.g. child/healthy adult/infirm person
- Did this affect their ability to escape the fire and thus affect the eventual outcome?
- Did the deceased die at the scene – or after removal from the scene? E.g. to hospital

5.05.3 The person reporting the fire

- Did this person have an official capacity or a duty of care towards the deceased?

5.05.4 The body

- Are there any signs that the deceased was restrained prior to the fire?
- Is the position of the body consistent with the history given?
- How much remains of the deceased?
- Consider the evidence of burning (or not) on the body (family will ask)
- What clothing remains on the deceased?

5.05.5 The scene

The local fire service report will probably cover all of the below which should be acceptable to the Coroner. However the CI will want to get a grasp of the information to be able to update the Coroner early, until the fire report comes in many weeks or months down the line.

- Describe the structure/building e.g.: public building/hotel/motel/barn/ garage/business premises/family home etc
- Of what is the structure/building made? E.g. brick/stone/concrete/metal/ wood etc

- What is the perceived cause of the fire? E.g. solvents/inflammables/ cooking/gas/cigarettes/candles
- Did the fire consume the immediate area where the deceased was lying?
- Is there any evidence of anything untoward at the scene? E.g. evidence of an assault prior to the fire
- Were there any fire alarms in the structure? Were they working? When were they last tested? (consider possibility of Health and Safety involvement or police corporate manslaughter charges if at place of work or care)
- Were there any smoke alarms in the structure? Were they working? When were they last tested? (consider possibility of Health and Safety involvement or police corporate manslaughter charges if at place of work or care)
- Where did the fire start – indoors/outdoors? In which room?
- Was there any evidence of smoking materials/alcohol containers/ medication containers/narcotics found at scene?
- Is there any indication of a suicide note or other paraphernalia at the scene?

5.05.6 Circumstances

- What were the activities of the deceased prior to the fire? E.g. smoking/ party/drinking

5.05.7 The event

- Was the event witnessed?
- Did others die or receive injuries as a result of this incident?
- Was there any rescue attempt?

5.05.8 Actions

- When body is removed pay careful attention to any personal property that may assist in identification of the body
- Leave any jewellery on body
- Note precise position of body – and if more than one their location in respect of the other(s) and tag as appropriate

5.05.9 Statements

The local fire service statements will usually be acceptable to a Coroner and there will be no need to duplicate these enquiries. However there may be circumstances – where the fire service is investigating itself for example – when this would not be adequate and a greater degree of involvement would be required.

If a matter is not suspicious the fire service report will form part of the evidence before the Coroner. However the CI will have to take other statements. For example, an elderly man living alone in his house accidentally setting fire to the house and being the only person to die in the process. Such a case will not require many police or fire service resources once the initial assessment has been made. Background statements from family and next of kin, neighbours etc as to habit and failing ability will fall to the CI.

5.06 Electrical deaths

5.06.1 The deceased
- Would this person be familiar with electricity? E.g. through work or hobby
- Would this person have been familiar with the particular equipment?

5.06.2 The body
- Where on body was deceased in contact with the apparatus?
- Are there burn marks on the body? Where? Photograph
- What clothing is the deceased wearing? Describe – particularly footwear
- Are there any burn / scorch marks on the clothing? Describe, photograph

"fatal electrocution may occur with no skin mark whatsoever, making the diagnosis entirely dependent upon the circumstances of the death." (Saukko and Knight 2004)

5.06.3 The finder
- What action did they take? E.g. disconnect power supply

5.06.4 Circumstances

- Was this an incident involving work? If yes involve HSE immediately (see 5.08 below) and while at scene if not already aware
- Was deceased using any electrical apparatus?
- Describe apparatus – new / used? Connection to power supply e.g. 3 pin plug/shaver
- Was an extension lead used?
- Did this occur indoor or outdoors?
- Circuit breaker? Describe location, type – was it bypassed?
- Has there been any attempt at resuscitation? E.g. by ambulance staff, which could have included intravenous cannulation. If so what sites and how many attempts?

"The severity of tissue damage 'including death' is directly related to a number of physical factors, which include current, voltage, resistance and time. For biological damage to occur, the body must be incorporated into an electrical circuit, so that there is a passage of electrons through the tissues." (Saukko and Knight 2004)

5.06.5 The scene (where found)

5.06.5.1 Indoors

- Type of floor e.g. metal/concrete/wood/other
- Condition of floor – dry/wet/other – describe

5.06.5.2 Outdoors

- Where is the power source coming from?
- What were the weather conditions - is it damp or wet? Was it at the probable time of the system?

5.06.6 The event

- Was the event witnessed? Clarify
- Did anyone try and rescue the deceased? Explain

5.06.7 Actions

- Call for electricity board to trace fault source (and satisfy that premises are safe for other occupants/users)
- Once electrical equipment made safe – seize it. Think chain of evidence
- Is the apparatus still usable? Take expert advice
- Has anyone previously been injured / killed from this same equipment or source prior to this incident?
- Arrange alcohol and toxicology tests on deceased

5.06.8 Additional statements

- Electricity supply company as to the supply – safe? Tampered with?
- Electricity company that attended (if different) will normally provide a full report covering their findings (including photographs) for the Coroner

5.07 Child deaths

5.07.1 Introduction

There is a multitude of literature available and articles in the medical journals on the issues surrounding child deaths. A number of cases over recent years have brought these issues clearly into the public arena. One publication worthy of note to all CIs is a report published in September 2004 entitled "Sudden unexpected death in infancy: the report of a working group convened by The Royal College of Pathologists and The Royal College of Paediatric and Child Health". This report can be accessed on the websites of either of the Royal Colleges: www.rcpath.org.uk and www.rcpch.ac.uk. It also contains a number of references for further reading in its reference section. This report is hereafter referred to as the SUDI report (2004). Legislation arose out of the SUDI report (see below).

Some Coroners now require that the death of any child under the age of 18 is referred to them. Under the Coroners (Amendment) Rules 2008 if the Coroner decides to order a post mortem examination report or to hold an inquest into the child's death, he must notify the Local Safeguarding Children Board (LSCB) of that child death within three working days. The LSCB is required to undertake child death review processes and supplies a report to the Coroner within 28 days of the death.

The Children Act 2004 is the primary and underpinning legislation of note. Arising out of that act, LSCBs became compulsory from April 2008. Prior to that there were pilot schemes around England and Wales. In some areas CIs are quite involved with the LSCB and the review process. In other areas there is only contact when a child has died.

A child death is any death up to the age of 18. However there is quite a difference between the 15 year old who collapses suddenly on the football pitch, and the four month old baby who is found dead in his / her cot.

Sudden Unexplained Death in Infancy (SUDI) usually refers to the death of babies and infants where the pathologist's cause of death after a post mortem examination is of Sudden Unexplained Death in Infancy (SUDI).

The Foundation for the Study of Infant Deaths (FSID) has published various documents to assist police forces and CIs when dealing with the sudden death of an infant. One such document is: "Sudden unexpected deaths in infancy: A suggested approach for police and Coroner's Officers". It is not repeated here but is recommended as a useful guide and is available to download as a pdf from their website www.fsid.org.uk.

In addition there is a document entitled "Recommendations for a joint agency protocol for the management of sudden unexpected deaths in infancy" available to download as a pdf from their website www.fsid.org.uk. This states that:

"When a person dies unexpectedly, the death must immediately be reported to the coroner by the doctor who decides the child has died, and the coroner then has jurisdiction over the body and everything pertaining to it. The coroner must therefore be involved in the development of the protocol, and his approval must be obtained for all items that lie within his jurisdiction.

The protocol should ensure that the following measures occur following any unexpected childhood death:

1. A rapid response to all unexpected child deaths *(sic)*

1. *Immediate notification of the death to the coroner (or his officer) (op cit)*

It further suggests that the role of the Coroner's Officer includes:

- *visit the family as necessary, keeping them fully informed about all the procedures that are taking place, and helping them with the practical arrangements.*
- *Liaise with involved professionals to gather and collate information for the coroner*
- *Inform front line professionals of the progress and outcome of the coronial inquiry*

The Child Bereavement Charity (CBC) (which was the Child Bereavement Trust until October 2007) has also published many leaflets, practice guidances, videos, DVDs and runs workshops and training. There is a web-based forum as well. Visit their website www.childbereavement.org.uk

OFSTED: OFfice for STandards in EDucation, children's services and skills has a role in relation to children as regards inspection and regulation. Visit www.ofsted.gov.uk for their inspection reports.

5.07.2 Police involvement

These deaths will attract intense initial police investigation and supervisory detective attendance. Each police force will have a policy in place guiding officers how to deal with child deaths. While the incidence of child murder is thankfully rare, it is a possibility that has to be considered in every case. There needs to be a balance with the acknowledged needs of the parents to grieve.

5.07.3 The CI's role

The role of the CI in a child death is not so much that of an investigative role, but rather more of a liaison and co-ordinating role. It will vary according to whether it is a suspicious case or not. If it is, then the CI's role is as outlined in Chapter 1.

The police will carry out an in-depth investigation into any child death, whether suspicious or not. This investigation will usually satisfy the Coroner if the matter comes to inquest, as in any other suspicious death which is later found not to be suspicious, and is downgraded (see section 1.15.1 above).

In a "non-suspicious child death", the CI's role is still more of a liaison / co-ordinating role. The importance and knowledge of the CI in these cases is acknowledged in the FSID document: "Sudden unexpected deaths in infancy: A suggested approach for police and Coroner's Officers". There some possible additional involvement of the CIs is envisaged as including:

- Visit the home of the family concerned
- Obtain medical records from all appropriate locations
- Liaise regarding the pathologist – should it be a paediatric, a forensic, both or a dually qualified forensic paediatric pathologist?
- Advise the family on any questions relating to the post mortem, seeing the baby, obtaining mementoes (foot and hand prints, hair locks, photographs etc)

"When a child dies unexpectedly, a paediatrician (on call or designated) should initiate an immediate information sharing and planning discussion between the lead agencies (i.e. health, police, LA children's social care) to decide what should happen next and who will do what. This will also include the coroner's officer."
(Working together to safeguard children section 7.35)

The SUDI report (2004) contains a section suggesting a summary of tasks of individual agencies and professionals, including Coroner's Officers.

The Confidential Enquiry into Maternal and Child Health published a report in May 2008: "Why Children Die: A Pilot Study (2006)" which also touches upon the role of Coroner's Officer and Coroner and includes a Coroner's perspective. It is available to buy through their website: www.cemach.org.uk

5.08 Deaths involving Health and Safety Executive (HSE) Investigations

5.08.1 The legal basis

Section 18 of the Health and Safety at Work etc Act 1974 make the HSE and local authorities responsible for making adequate arrangements for the enforcement of health and safety legislation with a view to securing the health, safety and welfare of workers and protecting others, principally the public. Visit www.hse.gov.uk for further information. HSE provides an Enforcement Guide for its inspectors, which is a publicly available document, setting out guidance for inspectors on investigating and prosecuting breaches of health and safety law.

See www.hse.gov.uk/enforce/enforcementguide/wrdeaths

5.08.2 Agreed protocol

There is a protocol agreed (since 1998, updated 2003) by ACPO, HSE, CPS, BTP and the LGA covering work related deaths. It is available to download from the HSE website: www.hse.gov.uk. A "work related death" is described in the protocol as:

"A fatality resulting from an incident arising out of or in connection with work." (Work-Related Deaths: A Protocol for Liaison 2003)

The introduction to the 2003 protocol states:

"This protocol has been agreed between the Health and Safety Executive (HSE), the Association of Chief Police Officers (ACPO), the British Transport Police (BTP), the Local Government Association and the Crown Prosecution Service (CPS). It sets out the principles for effective liaison between the parties in relation to work-related deaths in England and Wales, and is available to the public. In particular, it deals with incidents where, following a death, evidence indicates that a serious criminal offence other than a health and safety offence may have been committed. The protocol addresses issues concerning general liaison and is not intended to cover the operational practices of the signatory organisations." (Work-Related Deaths: A Protocol for Liaison 2003)

HSE, local authorities, the police and the CPS have different roles and responsibilities in relation to a work-related death.

Additionally there is a Memorandum of Understanding (MOU) between the Coroners Society of England and Wales (CSEW) and the HSE (2007) which "is intended to promote and continue effective working relationships between Coroners and HM Inspectors of Health and Safety." It is "a voluntary agreement". It is "not binding and is not intended to create any legally enforceable rights, obligations or restrictions".

CIs should have a copy of this document which is available to download from the HSE website, and should refer to it whenever there is a death involving HSE:

"It is envisaged that there will be discussions between the Coroner (or the Coroner's Officer) and the HSE inspector to ascertain whether there is any concern regarding the disclosure of any documents." (Memorandum of Understanding between the Coroners' Society England and Wales and the Health and Safety Executive 2007)

5.08.3 Prosecutions

The police investigate serious criminal offences such as manslaughter. The CPS decides whether such a case will proceed to court.

HSE prosecute health and safety offences. Sometimes this may be the local authority or other enforcing authority as responsibility for health and safety falls under a number of different agencies. The CPS may also occasionally prosecute health and safety offences. Where the CPS has reviewed a case and decided not to prosecute, HSE, the local authority or other enforcing authority will usually await the result of the Coroner's inquest before charging any Health and Safety offences, unless waiting would prejudice the case.

5.08.4 Investigations

The police may take an early lead in these cases. Investigations may be carried out by the HSE or other agencies. However there may be cases where the HSE are reluctant to release the outcome of their investigations prior to the inquest. In other cases they may release their report to the Coroner with a strict embargo on disclosure by the Coroner.

5.08.5 The CI's role

With deaths involving Health and Safety investigations the CI's role is less directly investigative – perhaps especially where there are technical issues that may be beyond that CI's abilities. Instead it involves:

- Scene and investigation management
- Early agreement as to who investigates what
- Avoidance of multiple interviews of witnesses
- Co-ordination and liaison
- Dealing with disclosure issues
- Ensuring one liaison point for the bereaved, witnesses and other interested parties

The HSE has a number of useful publications on its website www.hse.gov.uk. Some of these relate specifically to deaths. Additionally there is one on infectious risks from human remains. See section 5.02.11 above on road deaths for the interaction between HSE and road traffic deaths.

5.08.6 Jury inquest?

The question of whether a jury is required or not is a difficult one and one easily left to the Coroner who will advise their officer appropriately in each case.

5.08.7 Corporate manslaughter

The issue of corporate manslaughter is another area where the police will be involved. The introduction of the Corporate Manslaughter and Corporate Homicide Act 2007 has provided a definition of the offence and parameters as to when the offence will be committed. To some extent this has made it easier for police to investigate and refer to CPS for a decision.

If it transpires that a case of corporate manslaughter is to be made by the CPS there may well be no full inquest hearing (Coroners Act 1988 section 16 (1) which will be covered in the Coroners and Justice Bill 2008 the adjournment is referred to as "suspension" under Chapter 1 section 14 and Schedule 1).

5.09 Deaths overseas: the Foreign and Commonwealth Office (F&CO)

Whenever there is a death overseas and the body comes to lie in a Coroner's jurisdiction, section 8 of the Coroners Act 1988 is applied. Where an inquest arises, the investigation will involve contact with the Foreign and Commonwealth Office (F&CO). A request should be made for all police evidence, photographs, plans, and medical evidence from the overseas country. This usually takes a number of months or longer to arrive, if it arrives at all. Every effort should be made to obtain it in order to assist the Coroner:

"......to ensure that the relevant facts are fully, fairly and fearlessly investigated" R v HM Coroner for North Humberside ex parte Jamieson (1995)

While waiting for the F&CO to assist in the retrieval of information from overseas, the CI will of course be able to obtain evidence by contacting witnesses direct, in the usual way. Even if such witnesses are overseas, emails can assist in this process.

Further information can be found on the F&CO Travel website at http://www.fco.gov.uk/travel. They have a leaflet: "Death Overseas" which can be downloaded from the "Our Publications" pages.

6

DEATHS IN CUSTODY

6.01 Introduction

6.01.1 The legal underpinning

The Coroners Act 1988 section 8(1) states that:

"Where a coroner is informed that the body of a person ("the deceased") is lying within his district and there is reasonable cause to suspect that the deceased:-
(c) has died in prison.. then ... the coroner shall as soon as practicable hold an inquest into the death of the deceased ..."

6.01.2 The nature of the death itself

Each death should be investigated according to the nature of the death itself. If "suspicious" then it should be treated as such. Any criminal investigation will take priority over any other e.g. prison, healthcare trust or Coroner's investigation if a death is one considered as "suspicious" (see Chapter 1).

This chapter considers therefore not the circumstances of the death itself so much as the proximity of the detaining organisations to the death.

6.01.3 Multiplicity of investigations

Staff in any organisation may resent being "interviewed" more than once about their involvement in the matter. Multiplicity of investigations is something that support groups and counsellors amongst others would seek to reduce. Indeed, anyone with compassion would wish to reduce the impact that such multiple interviews can cause. However, there are some occasions when multiplicity is inevitable and right and proper. The sorts of death discussed in this chapter fall into that category.

Staff may not take too readily to the presence of the CI at this time. There may be a view that the CI "does not understand the system" of the particular organisation and could therefore be prejudiced. Inter-personal skills of a CI therefore are needed when investigating deaths involving organisations more so than in many other deaths. This is to explain clearly and empathetically the role of the Coroner in a death, and thus the role of the CI in that place. They are also needed to ensure that the CI gains a full understanding – of the organisation itself and the hierarchies within it. (See also section 6.02.2 below.)

6.01.4 Commonality across investigations within other organisations

Most of the observations and suggestions in this chapter apply equally to deaths in prisons, police detention, mental institutions and healthcare settings. These are all large organisations that will carry out their own internal enquiry into any unexpected and potentially untoward death. They are also all organisations that may dislike feeling under scrutiny. (See also Chapters 9, 10, 11 and 12 for Deaths in Healthcare Settings).

6.01.5 Jury inquest

The government's position paper (2004) states:

*"We believe that there is real value in holding a judicial inquest. This allows the death to be publicly investigated by a local coroner in a court setting. Two types of death might be **referred to the coroner** (sic): those from a list of reportable cases .... see sample list at Annex 2)." (op cit paragraph 39)*

Annex 2 includes:

"Any death of a person detained in a prison or in military detention, in police custody, in a special hospital or under statutory mental health powers, or of a person resident in a bail or asylum hostel."

All deaths in custody / detention will lead to an inquest with a jury unless the matter is adjourned under section 16 Coroners Act 1988 as someone is brought to Crown Court e.g. on a murder / manslaughter / assisted suicide charge for the matter. In the Coroners and Justice Bill the adjournment is referred to as "suspension" under Chapter 1 section 14 and Schedule 1 Part 1. Even if this does happen there may still be a full inquest hearing if the inquest needs to be resumed. An example of when this might happen would be if the "defendant" dies before the trial takes place. In the Coroners and Justice Bill the circumstances of resumption are covered under Schedule Part 2.

The government's position paper (2004) discusses juries briefly:

"We believe the existing basis for using juries should continue. Broadly-speaking, juries are required where a death raises issues of broad public interest or confidence, for example a prison death, or where key facts are disputed." (op cit paragraph 73)

6.01.6 Article 2 compliant investigation
Article 2 of the Human Rights Act 1988 states:

"Everyone's right to life shall be protected by law. No one shall be deprived of his life intentionally save in the execution of a sentence of a court following his conviction of a crime for which this penalty is provided by law."

The requirement for an Article 2 compliant investigation in any death in custody or detention, including patients detained under the provisions of the Mental Heath Act, entails a much more thorough investigation. Such an investigation is demanding and time-consuming. This is because it has to examine not only 'how' and 'by what means' the deceased came by his death but also the circumstances of the death. The scope of the investigation of the circumstances of the death varies on a case by case basis.

In each case systems will need to be examined in depth to establish:

- What protocols, procedures and systems there were in the institution
- Were they adequate?
- Were the conditions, actions and circumstances at the time in accordance with those protocols, procedures and systems?
- Was there any failure of a system?
- Was there any failure of an individual?

Consequently, what comes within the scope of such an investigation may include:

- Whether or not it was appreciated that the harm, self or otherwise, was a real and immediate risk
- The adequacy of relevant protocols
- Completeness of documentation
- What information was available to the authorities
- What information was handed over by staff at each shift handover
- What information was available to the staff on duty at the time of the incident
- What was known or ought to have been known;
- Who should have taken what actions
- What training staff have had, how often, how recently
- What else was happening in that part of the institution at the time, or if relevant in other areas of the institution, that may have had an effect upon the circumstances of this death

Article 2 has been interpreted by the Courts as requiring the state to take positive steps to safeguard the lives of those in the UK.

An Article 2 enquiry needs to examine the cause(s) of death; any reasonably practicable steps (if any) that could have been taken and were not taken to prevent the death; and the precautions (if any) that ought to be taken to avoid or reduce the risk to others. The inquest may consider whether there are any reasonably practicable steps that could be taken to prevent any such deaths in the future.

The State is required to adopt safeguards that are practical and effective to ensure that the rights of persons within its jurisdiction are respected.

Any Article 2 inquest will inevitably result in a hearing where the Coroner sits with a jury. In such an inquest the jury's factual findings should be broad enough to achieve the aims of the inquest which include:

"to ensure so far as possible that the full facts are brought to light; that culpable and discreditable conduct is exposed and brought to public notice; that suspicion of deliberate wrongdoing (if unjustified) is allayed; that dangerous practices and procedures are rectified; and that those who have lost their relative may at least have the satisfaction of knowing that lessons learned from his death may save the lives of others". See the stated of case re Amin (2003)

The argument for a "specialist investigator" for any deaths where Article 2 is invoked is strengthened as the lack of understanding of the systems can lead to an incomplete investigation. (See also sections 5.01.2 above and 6.02.1 below)

6.02 Deaths in Her Majesty's Prison establishments

6.02.1 Prison investigations
From 1 April 2004 the Prisons and Probation Ombudsman (PPO) became responsible for investigating all deaths of prisoners and residents of probation hostels and immigration detention accommodation.

The introduction to the Prisons and Probation Ombudsman page on the website states:

"The Prisons and Probation Ombudsman investigates complaints from prisoners, those on probation and those held in immigration removal centres. He also investigates all deaths that occur among prisoners, immigration detainees and the

residents of probation hostels (Approved Premises)." www.ppo.gov.uk

See www.ppo.gov.uk for more information. If the website is followed through its links there is a section "Investigating fatal incidents". On this page it states:

"We investigate all deaths that occur in prison or young offender institutions, probation approved premises (often known as hostels), and immigration removal centres, whatever the cause of death. Sometimes, we also investigate the death of someone recently released from custody. Some people may have died of natural causes; others may have taken their own life, while for some the cause of death may initially be unknown. Our investigation tries to provide answers to family and friends about what happened. If failings are found, recommendations for improvements are made. After each investigation we produce an anonymised report which you can view in the Publications section." www.ppo.gov.uk

There are further sections on the PPO website about what they will do, which includes appointing their own FLO. This will be as well as the Prison Service appointed FLO and in some cases the police appointed FLO. Thus a prisoner's family may have three separate FLOs attached to liaise with them, as well as the CI.

All the premises described to above will be referred to in this chapter as "prisons" for ease.

Investigations by the PPO may not alone be acceptable to the Coroner. The need to carry out an independent investigation into the death and to be seen to do so requires an intensive investigation on behalf of the Coroner. Accordingly one role of the CI is to supply the independent investigation for the public at large and the family of the deceased in particular.

The extra inter-personal skills of the CI are needed to ensure that they have a full understanding – of the prison itself; of the particular wing(s) in the prison involved; of the regimes and routines that have been in place throughout the prisoner's stay within the prison service and that may have some bearing on the specific death. This information and expertise is built up through dealing with cases. There is an argument for "specialist" CIs to deal with certain types of deaths. This was considered in sections 5.01.2 and 6.01.6 above.

Prison deaths and deaths in any sort of custody / detention are one category where knowledge and expertise is invaluable and where the argument stands very strong - albeit not specifically cited in either of the two reports. The ability of a CI who knows the workings of the system concerned to properly investigate a death as described in this chapter far outstrips that of a novice CI.

6.02.2 Early intervention by the CI

Early involvement in the matter is vital. Arrangements should be made in advance of any such death between the prison and the local Coroner so that the prison hierarchy understand the coronial position and are less likely to resent it as an intrusion.

It is important not to feel intimidated by the prison involvement, nor by the large number of senior prison officials who will need to be seen. As the Coroner's investigation will inevitably be duplicative to the PPO investigation and indeed any reports that the prison staff may have supplied immediately post-incident, this is a situation where the prison staff may feel as if they are repeating the information. However it is the author's experience that strikingly different questions will be asked by the CI than by the PPO. Patience and understanding of the staff's predicament is therefore called for.

6.02.3 Specific investigation guidelines – over and above the generic checklist

6.02.3.1 The deceased (inmate)

- The previous medical and psychiatric history is going to assume a greater importance in prison deaths in case of any effect on the deceased and/or his/her state of health
- Why was this person detained here?
- What was the alleged crime? Were they on remand or have they been convicted?

- Have they been in prison/detention before?
- What was their nationality/ethnicity and their understanding of the English language and the British prison system?
- With whom had there been recent contact?
- What opportunities had there been to access drugs?

6.02.3.2 The deceased (visitor)

- Who was this person visiting?
- What were their movements from arriving at the front gate to the point of death?
- With whom had they had contact?
- What was their nationality/ethnicity and their understanding of the English language and the British prison system?
- With whom had there been recent contact?
- Might they have been carrying drugs to pass to an inmate and something gone wrong?

6.02.3.3 The finder

- Was this a prison officer or another detainee?
- Why was this person in the location so as to be able to find the deceased?
- If another detainee, how long had they known the deceased?

6.02.3.4 The body

- Extra attention needs to be paid to the possibility of marks that do not fit in with the account given – especially if the deceased was in a shared cell

6.02.3.5 The scene where found

- Was this in a prison? Category A/B/C/D prison? If not, what was the nature of the premises and detention?
- If within a prison: What wing? A young offender's wing/the Health Care Centre/the remand wing/the first night centre/the induction wing
- Was there CCTV of the cell / area?
- Or was this in a court while under care of private company working for prison service?
- Or was this in a "prison" vehicle?

6.02.3.6 Circumstances

- What was the time lapse between the most recent court appearance - for sentence or remand and the death? Days/weeks/hours
- Was there anyone else in the cell with the deceased? If yes treat as a suspect until proven otherwise to satisfaction of police and CI
- Had there been a recent change in circumstances for the deceased? E.g. a visit from family or solicitor/a recent court appearance/a change of status: remand to convicted/a recent bereavement of a family member/friend
- Is there an immediate impending court appearance?
- Has there recently been another death in the same establishment?
- What else was happening on that wing and in the prison at that time?
- Was there under-staffing? Why? (eg sickness, work to rule)
- Were there many other prisoners on ACCT system? How many? Was this an unusually high number?
- Has there been any restraint by prison officers? Why? What was the restraint method?

6.02.3.7 The event

- Was the event witnessed?
- Who by?
- What attempt did the witness make to prevent the death?
- If none – why none?
- If prevention was attempted – why was it unsuccessful?
- Was there any resuscitation attempt? Describe

6.02.3.8 The time

- If the event was witnessed - when did it occur?
- If the event was not witnessed – when was the deceased last seen alive? Times in prisons can usually be pinpointed fairly closely – although less so at night

6.02.3.9 Other considerations

- Is there any indication of a suicide note? Where? Is it in deceased's handwriting?

- If yes. Where and when was the paper and pencil supplied?
- Is there anything unusual to suggest anything other than a suicide or an accident?
- How does the death appear to have occurred?
- Does the death appear on the surface to be natural or unnatural?
- Does this appear to be a natural death unfortunately in prison?
- Does it appear to be a suicide or murder?
- The answer to these questions will have some bearing on the progress of the investigation

6.02.3.10 Actions

- Look for evidence to prove or disprove every possible explanation
- Look for suicide note(s)
- Take photographs of everything
- Search cell thoroughly for notes: under bedding under/in mattress; in bed/ chair/table legs; in toilet, outside window
- If there was CCTV - seize any recording. The SIO and the Coroner will both want to see it. Confer with Coroner as to acceptability of this and making copies of video. First check the clock or timing mechanism on the machinery and compare it with actual time for accuracy
- Look for implements used in the death
- Look at all prison documentation and obtain copies immediately. This will vary in each case but may include amongst others:
  core records; ACCT (Assessment Care in Custody and Teamwork) forms; warrants; medical forms showing initial assessment, subsequent consultations, nurses' interactions, doctors' sessions; use of force and/or restraint policy; visit order forms; records and transcripts of telephone calls made
- Photograph cell and place of death if different; photograph ligature point if applicable. Photograph ligature where attached to fixing point; photograph ligature in relation to the body. Seize ligature or plastic bag or sharp implement used. If ligature send to mortuary
- Ensure toxicology and alcohol screen is carried out in addition to any post mortem examination

- See if any post has been sent out by the deceased. Has it gone? Where to? If not – seize it from outgoing post bag
- If any telephone calls were made obtain a recording of the calls (all calls are recorded except Samaritans etc)
- Was the inmate self-medicating? Obtain full details and check for medications in the cell
- Consider obtaining copies of relevant training records of staff

6.02.3.11 Additional statements

- Should be obtained from any others detained in neighbouring cells or within the cell if multi-occupancy and not a suspect, whether negative or positive information is obtained. These should be obtained quickly as the prison population moves around frequently and the detainee may have moved elsewhere
- Should be obtained from anybody who came into contact with the deceased at any time along his prison journey (if relatively short) or most frequently in contact if in detention for a longer time
- A copy of the PPO report should be obtained as soon as it is available. Often there is an initial report with a fuller report some weeks or months later. Both should be obtained where this applies. The PPO has a good liaison with most Coroners and will usually release their report and then discuss issues of disclosure with the Coroner

6.03 Deaths in police detention or care

The government's position paper (2004) states:

*"We believe that there is real value in holding a judicial inquest. This allows the death to be publicly investigated by a local coroner in a court setting. Two types of death might be **referred to the coroner** (sic): those from a list of reportable cases .... see sample list at Annex 2)." (op cit paragraph 39)*

Annex 2 includes:

"Any death of a person detained in police custody."

6.03.1 Definition

Home Office Circular 13/2002 and section 118(2) of the Police and Criminal Evidence Act 1984, provide the definition of a death in police detention or care.

The Circular introduced four specific categories covering deaths of members of the public during or following contact with the police

The definition is divided into categories and this affects the level of police involvement – the higher the category the higher ranking the SIO will be and the more resources will be invested.

6.03.1.1 Category 1 Fatal road traffic incidents involving the police

This will include people who die in road accidents whilst attempting to avoid arrest and people who die in road traffic incidents involving the police.

Annex A of the Circular states that this definition covers all deaths of members of the public resulting from road traffic incidents involving the police, both where the person who dies is in a vehicle and where they are on foot.

6.03.1.2 Category 2 Fatal shooting incidents involving the police

This will include only people who die where police officers fire the fatal shots.

6.03.1.3 Category 3 Deaths in or following police custody

This will include people who die who have been arrested or otherwise detained by the police and deaths occurring while a person is being arrested or taken into detention.

Annex A of the Circular states that the death may have taken place on police, private or medical premises, in a public place or in a police or other vehicle.

Deaths in the following circumstances are amongst those covered by the definition:

• Where the person dies in or on the way to hospital (or some other medical premises) following or during transfer from police detention

- Where the person dies after leaving police detention and there is a link between that detention and the death
- Where the person is being detained for the purposes of exercising a power to stop and search
- Where the death is of a child or young person detained for their own protection
- Where the person is in the care of the police having been detained under the Mental Health Act 1983
- Where the person is in police custody having been arrested by officers from a police force in Scotland exercising their powers of detention under section 137(2) of the Criminal Justice and Public Order Act 1994
- Where the person is in police custody having been arrested under section 3(5) of the Asylum and Immigration Appeals Act 1993
- Where the person is in police custody having been served a notice advising them of their detention under powers contained in the Immigration Act 1971
- Where the person is a convicted or remanded prisoner held in police cells on behalf of the Prison Service under the Imprisonment (Temporary Provisions) Act 1980

6.03.1.4 Category 4 Deaths during or following other types of contact with the police

This will include people who die during or after some form of contact with the police which did not amount to detention and there is a link between that contact and the death.

Examples given in Annex A of the Circular include:

- Where the person is actively attempting to evade arrest and the death occurs otherwise than as the result of a road traffic incident
- Where there is a siege situation, including where a person shoots himself, or another, whilst police are in attendance
- Where a person is present at a demonstration and is struck by a police baton and subsequently dies

Deaths which follow police contact but which are not linked to that contact would not be covered. For example:

- attending police stations as innocent visitors or witnesses who are not suspects
- Those which occur in a police vehicle which is being used as an ambulance to transport a dying person to hospital quickly, but not under the circumstances described under the category "Deaths in police custody" (sic)
- Those where police attend the scene of an incident where a person, who has not been detained, has received fatal injuries

Annex A of the Circular notes that

- The above categorisations cannot be considered completely exhaustive
- Cases will still have to be considered individually to decide whether and how they should be recorded
- The term "police" includes police civilians as well as police officers
- Deaths involving off-duty police personnel are not included

6.03.2 Investigations

The police will usually carry out their own investigations into these deaths. There is in every police force a Professional Standards Department (PSD) (by whatever name) which will investigate immediately. They will probably be notified of the death before the CI is.

In some instances another police force will very quickly be appointed to investigate – to provide a degree of perceived independence. This appointment may be at the request of the police force concerned or the Independent Police Complaints Commission (IPCC).

These investigations are not necessarily in and of themselves acceptable to the Coroner. The obvious concern would be whether there had been any muddying of the waters. Such cases however are always overseen by the IPCC to provide the degree of independence that the Coroner needs and might not otherwise get in a case of the police investigating themselves. The relevant PSD will liaise with the IPCC from a very early stage.

6.03.3 Independent Police Complaints Commission (IPCC)

The IPCC took over from the Police Complaints Authority in 2004. It was created as part of the Police Reform Act 2002. There is a useful website www.ipcc.gov.uk and it would be worthwhile for every CI to visit this. It is stated there that:

"The Independent Police Complaints Commission (IPCC) ... is a Non-Departmental Public Body (NDPB), funded by the Home Office, but by law entirely independent of the police, interest groups and political parties and whose decisions on cases are free from government involvement. We have a legal duty to oversee the whole of the police complaints system, created by the Police Reform Act 2002, our aim is to transform the way in which complaints against the police are handled." (www.ipcc.gov.uk)

The role of the CI is to supply the independence for the investigation that the police and to some extent the IPCC do not supply. It is also to ensure that all information made available to IPCC and PSD is also made available to the Coroner. This may not be accepted readily by the PSD or IPCC and this is a situation where antipathy to the CI may be quite high. Inter-personal skills therefore are needed more so than in many other deaths.

The possible variables of the circumstances of death in police detention are virtually as many as there are variable deaths; what can occur outside police detention can occur in police detention.

Each death should be investigated therefore according to the nature of the death itself. If suspicious then it should be treated as such. If not it will still require a full investigation. If someone dies of a heart attack in police detention, a full investigation is still required and there will still be a jury inquest. The jury may return a verdict of natural causes – but there will have been a full independent investigation into the circumstances surrounding the death.

This section of this chapter considers therefore not the circumstances of the death itself so much as the proximity of the police organisation to it.

6.03.4 Early intervention by the CI

Early involvement in the matter is vital. Arrangements should be made in advance of any such death between the police and the local Coroner so that the police hierarchy understand the coronial position and are less likely to resent it as an intrusion.

It is important not to feel intimidated by the police involvement, nor by the large number of senior officers who will want to be present, intervene and take control.

Equally it is important not to be too familiar with police – especially if they are current or former colleagues – as this can interfere with the impartiality that the Coroner - through his Investigator - is required to have.

6.03.5 Specific investigation guidelines – over and above the generic checklist

Many of these will be similar to a death in prison and the phrase "police officer" can often be substituted for "prison officer" in the section at 6.02 above. Similar questions will need to be asked of those in police detention as need to be asked of other prisoners above.

6.03.5.1 The deceased

- The previous medical and psychiatric history is going to assume a greater importance in police detention deaths in case of effect on the deceased and/or his/her state of health
- Did the person complain of any medical condition such that a police doctor was asked to attend? Did the doctor attend? If not why not?
- Why was this person detained on this occasion?
- Have they been in police detention before?
- What is their nationality/ethnicity and their understanding of the English language and the British police system?
- Were others detained by police at the same time for the same reason?

6.03.5.2 The finder

- Was this a police officer or some other within the environs of the police ambit?
- Why was this person in the location so as to be able to find the deceased?
- Was the finder the arresting or detaining officer?

6.03.5.3 The body

- Because of the justifiable use of force by police, particular attention will need to paid to any signs of restraint and the pathologist will need as much information as possible before starting the post mortem examination. Polaroid photographs will be invaluable in these cases

6.03.5.4 The scene where found

- Was this in a police station?
- If yes, exactly where in the police station was it?
- How does the death appear to have occurred?
- Does the death appear on the surface to be natural or unnatural?
- Does this appear to be a natural death unfortunately in a police station?
- Does it appear to be a suicide or murder?
- The answer to these questions will have some bearing on the progress of the investigation
- Look for implements used in the death
- Look at police documentation in relation to the deceased as early as possible

6.03.5.5 Circumstances

- What were the circumstances of the arrest?
- Was any force used in order to achieve the arrest?
- Were handcuffs* used?
- Were limb restraints** used?
- If limb restraints were used, have they previously been medically reviewed?
- Was incapacitant spray*** used?
- Was a police truncheon used?
- Was the use of any force witnessed by any non-police personnel?

- Was force necessary in the police station after the detention process had begun?
- Was any force used appropriate?
- What was the time lapse between the arrest / detention and the death?
- Was there anyone else in the cell with the deceased? If yes treat as a suspect until proven otherwise
- Was there anyone else in the police car en route to the police station?

In 2006 ACPO published a document entitled Guidance on the Use of Handcuffs. This is available to download from the ACPO website: www.acpo.police.uk.

The guidance comments about justification for use of handcuffs:

"Any intentional application of force to the person of another is an assault. The use of handcuffs amounts to such an assault and is unlawful unless it can be justified. Justification is achieved through establishing not only a legal right to use handcuffs, but also good objective grounds for doing so in order to show that what the officer or member of police staff did was a reasonable, necessary and proportionate use of force." (op cit)

The physical condition of the detained person is considered:

"The physical condition of a person is another consideration in deciding whether or not handcuffs should be applied or their application continued. For example, where a person has a condition that may be aggravated when handcuffed, this might make their use unreasonable. When handcuffs are used, the condition of the person should be monitored to ensure that there is no particulur risk of injury or death." (op cit)

** In 2006 ACPO published a document entitled Guidance on the Use of Limb Restraints. This is available to download from the ACPO website: www.acpo.police.uk.

It states:

"The term 'limb restraint' indicates a device that is designed and used to restrict the range of movement of the arms and / or legs. Its application should prevent a person from kicking and / or punching and allow for safe transportation of the person in a vehicle to a place of safety."

Additionally:

"Any device adopted should have been medically reviewed to minimise the potential of injury to the person. Reviews should also indicate the medical implications of protracted use and suggest time limits, where appropriate. This is particularly important if the device is to be used around the upper body or chest. Limb restraints should only be used by those officers who have received appropriate training." (op cit)

*** In 2006 ACPO published a document entitled Guidance on the Use of Incapacitant Spray. This is available to download from the ACPO website: www.acpo.police.uk .

Incapacitant spray includes CS spray and PAVA spray.

CS is described as:

"a peripheral sensory irritant. In most cases spraying will result in the subject's eyes being forced shut, a burning sensation on the skin around the eyes and face, when inhaled, their breathing may be affected. In most cases this action will be sufficient to render a subject incapable of continuing an attack. The effects may be instantaneous or can be delayed for up to 20 seconds."

PAVA is described:

"Irritant is dispensed from a hand held canister in a liquid stream that contains a 0.3% solution of PAVA (Pelargonic Acid Vanillylamide) in a solvent of aqueous ethanol. The propellant is nitrogen." (op cit)

PAVA affects the detained person in that it:

"primarily affects the eyes causing closure and severe pain. The pain to the eyes is reported to be greater than that caused by CS. The effectiveness rate is very high once PAVA gets into the eyes." (op cit)

Recovery after use of PAVA:

"Close monitoring of a subject throughout the recovery period is of utmost importance. If the individual experiences difficulties in resuming normal breathing then medical assistance must be sought immediately and must be given precedence over conveying the subject to the police station. Difficulties with breathing may be reflected in an individual displaying an audible wheeze or an inability to complete a sentence in one breath or an increased respiratory rate beyond the normal recovery period. The expected recovery period is 5 minutes after exposure. If the individual has been restrained either by hand or through the use of handcuffs or other restraint devices then particular attention should be given to monitoring their breathing." (op cit)

CIs should be aware of all of these documents and should provide the Coroner with a copy of the relevant document if a death involves police use of any of these methods of restraint.

6.03.5.6 The event
- Was the event witnessed?
- Who by?
- What attempt did the witness make to prevent the death?
- If none – why none?
- If prevention was attempted – why was it unsuccessful?
- Was there any resuscitation attempt – describe

6.03.5.7 The time
- Timings for someone in police detention can usually be pinpointed with a high degree of accuracy – although less so at night or once the detainee is

placed in the cell and awaiting the next part of the detention process. Even then there should never be a period of more than an hour for any detainee without being seen and checked

6.03.5.8 Other considerations

- vIs there any indication of a suicide note? Where? Is it in deceased's handwriting?
- If yes – where and when was the paper and pencil supplied?
- Is there anything unusual to suggest anything other than a suicide or an accident
- The police will usually want to assign an FLO. It is important to check with the family that they want this or accept it. If they do the CI should liaise with the FLO in the usual way whenever one is assigned
- If handcuffs were used, have the officer(s) been trained in their use? When were they trained?
- If limb restraints were used, have the officer(s) been trained in their use? When were they trained?
- If incapacitant spray was used, have the officer(s) been trained in its use? When were they trained?

6.03.5.9 Actions

- Look for evidence to prove or disprove every possible explanation
- Look for suicide note(s)
- Take photographs – separate from police Scientific Support Branch photographs to negate allegations of non-independence (unless being considered "suspicious" and to do so would contaminate the scene)
- Obtain CCTV of all actions within the police custody block and audio tapes if available
- Obtain copies of all police documentation immediately. This may include custody records, medical records, police pocket notebooks, investigator notebooks
- Obtain copies of any medical reviews of limb restraints
- Obtain copies of any training records in respect of limb restraints

6.03.5.10 Additional Statements

- From any others detained by the police in the same location or at the same time – whether negative or positive information is obtained
- From anybody who came into contact with the deceased at any time between the arrest / detention and the discovery of death. This may include police officers, police civilian staff, police doctor, custody centre staff
- A copy of the police enquiry report should be obtained as soon as it is available. The police will want to discuss issues of disclosure with the Coroner

CIs should also make themselves aware of the contents of the 2002 HO Circular on guidance to the police about pre-inquest disclosure following a death in police custody.

6.04 Deaths in mental institutions or where the deceased is detained under a section of the Mental Health Act 1983.

The government's position paper (2004) states:

*"We believe that there is real value in holding a judicial inquest. This allows the death to be publicly investigated by a local coroner in a court setting. Two types of death might be **referred to the coroner** (sic): those from a list of reportable cases .... see sample list at Annex 2)." (op cit paragraph 39)*

Annex 2 includes:

"Any death of a person detained in a special hospital or under statutory mental health powers."

6.04.1 Internal investigations

The Trust or institution will usually carry out their own internal investigation into such a death. They will want to do so as quickly as possible and may have an internal policy giving time scales. To do this they will want the person's medical notes. However the Coroner also wants those notes immediately. A Coroner will indeed want to see the outcome of any such internal enquiry but this will not be adequate in the way of an independent investigation on behalf of the Coroner.

The role of the CI and the need for an inquest at all is not always understood and may need careful and clear explanation, even to senior staff within the Trust or institution.

Inter-personal skills are needed more to explain the remit of the Coroner's inquest and attempt to allay any suspicions that staff may perceive.

The possible variables of the circumstances of death in such an institution are as variable as those outside such a place. Whilst there is an aim of preventing self harm and suicide the methodology tends not to be to lock someone in a fixture free environment with no clothes. It is rather that to try and address the causes of such feelings / actions and assist the individual to overcome them.

Each death should be investigated therefore according to the nature of the death itself. If suspicious then it should be treated as such.

This section considers therefore not the circumstances of the death itself so much as the duty of care in proximity to it.

6.04.2 Early intervention by the CI

Early involvement in the matter is vital. It is helpful if arrangements have been made in advance of any such death between the mental healthcare provider and the local Coroner so that there is a clear understanding of the role of the Coroner and staff. This is more likely to lead to a positive reaction from staff and therefore more information more readily given.

6.04.3 Specific investigation guidelines – over and above the generic checklist

6.04.3.1 The deceased

- The previous medical and psychiatric history is going to assume a greater importance in such deaths

- Has the person previously been detained under a Section?
- Is the person currently detained under section? Which? For how long?
- Is there any previous history of self-harm or suicide attempt?
- Is there any history of suicidal ideation?
- Had the person been assessed as regards a suicide risk?

6.04.3.2 The finder

- Was this person a member of staff or some other person?
- Why was this person in the location so as to be able to find the deceased?

6.04.3.3 The body

- Are there any marks of previous self-harm or suicide attempts?

6.04.3.4 The scene where found

- Was this in a secure location such as a secure wing?
- How does the death appear to have occurred?
- Does the death appear on the surface to be natural or unnatural?
- Does this appear to be a natural death?
- Does it appear to be a suicide or murder?
- The answer to these questions will have some bearing on the progress of the investigation
- Look for implements used in the death
- Look at all documentation – obtain copies immediately. This may involve removing them, taking away and copying and then returning to the Trust to assist them in their own enquiry

6.04.3.5 Circumstances

- What appears to have occurred and how?

6.04.3.6 The event

- Was the event witnessed?
- Who by?
- What attempt did the witness make to prevent the death?
- If none – why none?

- If prevention was attempted – why was it unsuccessful?
- Was there any resuscitation attempt – describe

6.04.3.7 The time

- What level of observation was in place for the deceased? Constant/every 15 minutes/every 30 minutes?
- Timings for someone under a section can usually be pinpointed with a high degree of accuracy – although perhaps less so at night

6.04.3.8 Other considerations

- Is there any indication of a suicide note? Where? Is it in deceased's handwriting?
- Is there anything unusual to suggest anything other than a suicide?
- If it appears to be an accident – how did it come about?
- Establish the identity of the Registered Medical Officer (RMO); Community Psychiatric Nurse (CPN); key worker
- Consider medication compliance issues – did the service user take their medication as prescribed or were there issues?

6.04.3.9 Actions

- Obtain copies of all risk assessments. How often were they done? Are they properly recorded?
- Obtain medication records and check for compliance and appropriate dosage
- Obtain copy of the Serious Untoward Incident (SUI) report
- Establish whether there have been any tribunals and when the last one was and the outcome of that process.
- Contact the deceased's solicitor or advocate within the Mental Health Review process and obtain a report from that advocate
- Download and print off relevant NICE Guidelines

6.04.3.10 Additional statements

- From any other patients or residents in the facility (so long as mentally competent) - whether negative or positive information is obtained

- A copy of the institution's internal report should be obtained as soon as it is available
- A report from the Consultant in charge of the overall treatment and care of the deceased will be needed as well as from any staff who had a close rapport with them as well as anyone on duty at the time
- A report from the RMO (especially if the deceased had been in the community under a supervision order
- A report from the key worker (who co-ordinates all the different aspects of care, to include whether there were any difficulties in obtaining the right support at the right time
- A report from any CPN involved

6.04.4 'Never events' and mental health

In March 2009 the National Patient Safety Agency (NPSA) National Reporting and Learning System (NRLS) issued a document: "Never events Framework 2009/10: Process and action for Primary Care Trusts 2009/10" which is available from the NPSA NRLS website (www.npsa.nhs.uk/nrls) to download in pdf format. The framework identifies an initial core list of eight "never events" which are defined as:

"serious, largely preventable patient safety incidents that should not occur if the available preventative measures have been implemented".

Events five and six on the core list of 'never events' would specifically apply if the 'event' had occurred in a mental health setting (see also section 9.05.2.1 below):

Event five on the core list refers to 'Inpatient suicide using non-collapsible rails' which is described as:

"Suicide using curtain or shower rails by an inpatient in an acute mental health setting."

The explanation in Appendix A of the framework document states:

"Inpatients in mental health units are at high risk of suicide, and hanging or strangulation is the most common method of suicide in this group"

Appendix A refers to various advice documents which CIs can access if the need arises. These include a NICE guideline (CG16) on self-harm which is of particular relevance and which can be downloaded from the NICE website www.nice.org.uk.

Event six on the core list refers to 'Escape from within the secure perimeter of medium or high secure mental health services by patients who are transferred prisoners' which is described as:

"A patient who is a transferred prisoner escaping from medium or high secure mental health services where they have been placed for treatment on a Home Office restriction order"

The explanation in Appendix A of the framework document is that this relates to:

"A patient who is a transferred prisoner escaping from medium or high secure mental health services where they have been placed for treatment on a Home Office restriction order..... Escape from secure mental health services is a high profile safety issue for other patients, staff and the public. Mental health providers should have local policies in place to define the security arrangements as per the document: 'Standards for Medium Secure Units, 2007' "

Appendix A refers to various advice documents which CIs can access if the need arises.

If such events should involve any death, the CI should ensure they take into account the 'never event' process that will be instigated. For more information on this see the document itself and also section 9.05.2.1 below.

Although the never events are perceived as likely to occur in a particular care setting they might occur in other care settings and if they do then CIs need to be aware that the never event reporting procedure should be followed.

6.0.5 Care Quality Commission (CQC)

The Care Quality Commission (CQC) was established under the Health and Social Care Act 2008 and came into existence on 1st October 2008.

From 1st April 2009 the CQC replaced the Commission for Social Care Inspection (CSCI), the Healthcare Commission and the Mental Health Act Commission (MHAC).

The CQC website www.cqc.org.uk links to the websites of these three organisations and its front page stated in April 2009:

"We regulate health and adult social care services, whether provided by the NHS, local authorities, private companies or voluntary organisations. And, we protect the rights of people detained under the Mental Health Act." www.cqc.org.uk

The rationale for a new organisation to replace the preceding three was stated on the CQC website:

"As the needs of people who use social care and health services, carers and their families have changed over the last decade, responsibility for social care and health services has come together.... Now the Care Quality Commisisons will be the first opportunity to brign these functions together under one iundependent regulator." www.cqc.org.uk

The CQC Chair Barbara Young stated at its launch on 1 April 2009:.

"CQC will join up the regulation of health and adult social care across the public and independent sectors for the first time.... Over the next three years we will bring a range of services, including primary care, GP and dental services into a single registration system spanning both the health and adult social care system." www.cqc.org.uk

On their website the CQC provides guidance for professionals working with people detained under the Mental Health Act. It also lists briefings for Mental Health Act commissioners giving additional guidance on, and or interpretation of, current aspects of the Mental Health Act. Certain forms are available to download from the site as well.

It is not yet clear what the changes will be as regards to the investigation of deaths in mental institutions that have been in place under the remit of the MHAC. However it is likely that it will have the same monitoring, regulatory and investigative powers. It is also likely that it will need to be informed of any inquest hearings into the deaths of people who died in a mental health institution. (See section 9.05.1 below for more about the CQC.)

6.06 Mental Health Act Commission (MHAC)

The front page of the MHAC stated in February 2009:

"From 1 April 2009 a new independent regulator of all health and adult social care in England comes into being. The Care Quality Commission will bring together the work of the CSCI and the Healthcare Commission and the Mental Health Act Commission in England. In Wales the duties of the Mental Health Act Commission will be taken over by Healthcare Inspectorate Wales,

The Care Quality Commission will champion the rights and interests of everyone who uses health and adult social care services in England. It will continue and build on the excellent work of CSCI, HCC and MHAC and have tough new powers to act on the public's behalf if services are unacceptably poor.

Integrating health and social care under a single regulator means that the Care Quality Commission can bring together the very best inspection and regulation methods and act as one port of call for independent information on standards, safety and available provision.

The Mental Health Act Commission wholeheartedly supports the Care Quality Commission in its ambition to ensure the safety and quality of health, mental health and social care services in England and to contribute to the long term achievement of ambitious standards of care."

7

DEATHS THROUGH INTOXICATION

7.01 Alcohol Related Deaths

7.01.1 Introduction

These may be due to "chronic alcoholism" where liver cirrhosis is often given as the most usual cause of death. These are no longer regarded as unnatural, although at one time they were. When a pathologist gives a cause of death as "chronic alcoholism" this will usually be regarded as natural by the Coroner and there will be no need for an inquest.

However, they may equally be due to "acute alcohol intoxication" with blood levels of ethanol, of 486mg/dL or more in blood not uncommon. These are not regarded as natural and will therefore result in an inquest. The CI should attend such deaths for reasons as outlined in Chapter 1.

7.01.2 Specific investigation guidelines – over and above the generic checklist

7.01.2.1 The deceased

- External appearance unkempt, lack of personal hygiene (not always)
- Alcohol related health problems (gastric ulcers etc)
- Evidence of jaundice
- Ascites (swelling of abdomen)
- Bruises (e.g. from old falls while drunk)
- History of alcohol consumption from friends and family
- Were they a regular drinker? If so did they binge or was it constant?
- History of other addiction e.g. drug abuse (the 2 often go together) from friends and family

- History of above from GPs or other professionals – social workers, psychiatric workers to include past treatment
- History of past attempts to "dry out" / detoxify with details of dates, frequency and level of success

7.01.2.2 The body

- Alcohol related deaths can raise alarm due to presence of injuries on the body. Are there any wounds on the body that are not consistent with known former injuries or current incident?
- Are there other marks that indicate what may have occurred? E.g. bruises from regularly falling over while drunk

7.01.2.3 The scene where found

- The scene – typically (but not always) disorganised, dirty, poor, unhygienic, cold (all indications that all available money is spent on alcohol)
- Direct evidence – alcohol containers – number
- Location – on display, in cupboards, in bins, in toilet cisterns, under bed, or other hiding places
- Type of drink - cheap & strong cider; vodka (lack of smell) are generic favourites, although some will have their favourite tipple (often whisky)
- Blood (evidence of oesophageal varices) often found in sink or basin or bucket/container by bed
- Melaena (faeces with blood) is often found in toilet, on mattress, in pyjamas/trousers/dressing gown
- Coffee ground haematemesis (evidence of older bleeding)

7.01.2.4 Circumstances

- Is there a known history of alcohol abuse/alcoholism? If not what occurred to cause this particular excessive drinking event?

7.01.2.5 Other considerations

- Is there any indication of alcohol or drugs paraphernalia or tablet bottles or packets? Where?
- Is there anything unusual to suggest anything other than a suicide or an accident?

7.01.2.6 Actions

- Take photographs of scene / home showing lifestyle
- Examine alcohol containers – how many: full / empty / part empty
- Note make of alcohol

7.01.2.7 Statements to be obtained

- Establish whether type of alcohol containers found fits with what the deceased usually drunk – e.g. strong cider/whisky/vodka. Often there is a particular drink always chosen and anything else would be out of the ordinary

It is not unusual for a CI to be asked by relatives or friends how much alcohol must have been consumed over what period of time for the person to have achieved an alcohol levels such as is found at post mortem examination. Caution is advised in giving any response to such a question.

"The most important statement in this respect is to stress the utter unreliability and inaccuracy of attempting back calculations in either direction. Only gross approximation can be achieved and no pretence at accuracy must be offered."
(Saukko and Knight 2004)

The safest words from the CI would be repetition of the above statement which was written by a forensic pathologist.

7.02 Drug Related Deaths

Where it is thought that death may have occurred due to an overdose of prescribed or over the counter medication the CI should attend.

It is rare that someone is forced to swallow large amounts of tablets against their will. However, the possibility of assisted suicide should always be considered. Is there a chance that the finder was involved in such a scenario? If this is possible then the police would need to be involved as the offence of aid and abet, counsel or procure suicide carries a maximum sentence of 14 years under the Suicide Act 1961. Overdose is a very usual method in such deaths, as it is in suicide pacts.

7.02.1 Prescribed drugs

It will help the pathologist and toxicologist to calculate how many tablets the deceased has taken by recording how many tablets were prescribed, the date of issue, how many should have been taken and how many remain.

Medications need to be accounted for and scheduled. The number of tablets missing, as against the number of tablets that should have been present provide useful information. This is very important, because toxicological analysis is of little help in these circumstances.

This will also assist the Coroner in the determination as to whether the overdose was in such a massive proportion that it is likely that death was intended.

The CI should take possession of any remaining tablets / capsules / liquid, containers empty or otherwise; and any other containers which included liquid or other substances that could have been ingested and contributed to death. The contents of all containers should be noted and details included in any information to the pathologist and toxicologist.

7.02.1.1 Drugs chart

See Appendix 4 for a sample drugs chart that can be used to methodically record the information required by the pathologist, toxicologist and the Coroner.

7.02.1.2 The deceased

- Is there a history of tablet overdose or mis-dose? Is it of this particular drug suspected on this occasion? If mis-dose obtain full evidence as to past incorrect dosage and times of taking tablets and confusion as to whether it has been taken or not
- Is there a history of alcohol or other substance abuse?

7.02.1.3 The finder

- Who found him? Is this person known to the deceased? What is their relationship?

7.02.1.4 The body

- Are there marks that indicate what may have occurred?
- Are there any signs that the tablets/liquid was forced into the deceased – marks/injury to the mouth, bruises on head, arms where restrained

7.02.1.5 The scene where found

- Is there evidence of tablet / liquid containers in the premises? If so precisely where? Or in the bins outside?
- If there is no evidence – who has cleaned up and why?

7.02.1.6 Circumstances

- Are there other medications unused still present? If so, list, photograph, seize
- Are there containers that may have been complementary (e.g. glasses or jugs or bottles that contained liquids to assist swallowing? If so, list, photograph, seize

7.02.1.7 The event

- Has there been any attempt at resuscitation? E.g. by ambulance staff – which could have included drugs of reversal that may affect toxicological test results?

7.02.1.8 Other considerations

- Prescribed medication belonging to other family members may have been taken and this needs to be considered

7.02.1.9 Actions

- Look for suicide note(s)
- Seize any potential evidence - e.g. syringes/drugs/tablets (or liquid form)/ repeat prescriptions/notes
- If there is a used syringe and/or needle near to the body consider sending to toxicology lab (in secure sharps container) to assist in toxicological analysis, if they will accept such evidence

7.02.1.10 Additional statements

- A GP report as to what medication was issued to the deceased, how much issued and when issued. Is there evidence of stockpiling?
- A report should be obtained for the senior police officer who attended to state how they satisfied themselves that this was not a suspicious death,

7.02.2 Illegal drugs

7.02.2.1 Offences

When a death has occurred that is believed to be due to illegal drugs by one route or another, the police will want to attend to ascertain if any offences can be detected. Such offences might include possession, or possession with intent to supply, or supplying – under the Misuse of Drugs Act 1971. The police interest in a death caused by illegal drugs generally extends no further than this, unless there is reason to suspect the drugs have been administered by someone else.

The Coroner will require a full investigation into any drugs related death. A CI then must ensure that drugs related deaths are investigated as fully as any other. The CI should attend all such deaths as well as the police.

7.02.2.2 Verdicts

A Coroner who uses short verdicts may need to consider whether a drug related death should be called "non-dependent drug abuse" or "dependence on drugs". To assist the Coroner in reaching a decision between these two verdicts the deceased's past and recent history in relation to drug and substance abuse must be evidenced.

7.02.2.3 Previous history

Such history might be demonstrable through previous convictions of the deceased stretching back over many years, depicting a clear history. However, absence of any previous conviction does not necessarily mean that there is no history of past abuse. Rather it might mean that the deceased has not come to the attention of the police.

DEATHS THROUGH INTOXICATION

Whether or not a Coroner is entitled to have sight of someone's previous convictions is a matter of separate debate, beyond this book. Whether or not a CI is allowed access to such information is also a matter that ought to be clarified elsewhere.

7.02.2.4 The deceased

- Is there a history of drug taking? Is it of this particular drug suspected on this occasion?
- Is there a history of past overdosage (although not fatal)
- Is the deceased believed to be a dealer?
- Is there a history of alcohol or other substance abuse?

7.02.2.5 The finder

- Who found him? Is this person known to the deceased? What is their relationship?
- Is this person a suspected drug user? Does this render their evidence less reliable?
- Is this person believed to be a dealer?

7.02.2.6 The body

- Is there any tourniquet? E.g. belt / shoelace
- Are there marks that indicate what may have occurred? E.g. bruises from regularly falling over while drunk; track marks indicative of an IV user
- Are there any signs that the intravenous was forced on the deceased – bruises on head, arms where restrained

7.02.2.7 The scene where found

- Is there evidence of drug use in the premises? E.g. needles/syringes/ methadone bottles/silver foil wraps/citric acid and other mixers/other drugs paraphernalia
- If there is no evidence – who has cleaned up and why?

7.02.2.8 Circumstances

- If on this occasion intravenous administration is suspected, was the site logical for self administration? E.g. the left antecubital fossa for a right handed person

- Are there other drugs unused still present? (prescribed or illegal). List, photograph, arrange for police to seize (or if we are authorised under future new laws, seize self)
- What route of administration is believed to have been used on this occasion – IV, oral, snorting, smoking

7.02.2.9 The event

- Has there been any attempt at resuscitation? E.g. by ambulance staff – which could have included intravenous cannulation? If so what sites and how many attempts?
- Was the event witnessed?
- Was the witness also using drugs? How come they are still alive?

7.02.2.10 The time

- It is rare to establish an exact time of death in drugs cases as there are not often coherent witnesses

7.02.2.11 Other considerations

- Prescribed medication belonging to other family members may have been taken and this needs to be considered

7.02.2.12 Actions

- Look for suicide note(s) – more likely with prescribed drugs than illegal
- Seize any potential evidence - e.g. syringes/drugs/tablets (or liquid form)/ repeat prescriptions/notes
- If there is a used syringe and/or needle near to the body send to toxicology lab (in secure sharps container) to assist in toxicological analysis

7.02.2.13 Additional statements

- A GP report or a report from a detoxification unit will be invaluable in the case of illegal drugs
- A report should be obtained for the senior police officer who attended to state not only how they satisfied themselves that this was not a suspicious death, but also any relevant information about the deceased's drug use

7.02.2.14 Documentation after inquest

Deaths due to drugs are monitored nationally and most Coroners or their Investigators will complete a form for the National Programme on Substance Abuse Deaths based at St George's Hospital Medical School in each such case. Completion of the form is entirely voluntary and not statutorily required. In some areas the form may be copied to the local police force drugs intelligence officer. CIs should ascertain in their individual areas whether it is they or their Coroner who submits this form. Either way the CI should ensure the answers to the questions on the form are established to assist with its accurate completion after the inquest.

7.02.3 Solvents

There is a similar scheme for reporting deaths by volatile substances – or solvents – to the Department of Public Health at St George's Hospital Medical School in London.

7.03 Death by water intoxication

7.03.1 Introduction

Intoxication is synonymous with poisoning. Human bodies need an appropriate balance of chemicals to work efficiently. Disturb that balance by any means and the body may die.

Water logging of the system can alter the sodium levels and the osmolality. This can cause death. It is quite rare for this to occur – generally speaking we do not drink too much water. Our natural instincts seem to protect us.

Certain mental disorders can reduce the natural self-protection mechanisms – such as dementia or schizophrenia. However, even so, such a death would be inquestable.

7.03.2 The deceased

- Build of deceased
- Any known medical condition that might predispose excess drinking? E.g. diabetes. Is there any history of it in the blood family?

- Any known mental condition that might predispose excess drinking? E.g. schizophrenia/dementia
- Any signs of an unknown mental condition that might predispose excess drinking?
- Where found? Date and time found? By whom found? In hospital or not?

7.03.3 The next of kin/family

- Who are the family members or next of kin?
- What can they tell us about deceased's behaviour – especially as regards drinking habits and recent changes?
- Might any of these people have been involved in the death and have a part to conceal?

7.03.4 The body

- Are there any wounds on the body that are not consistent with known former injuries or current incident?
- Are there any signs that the deceased was forced to drink excess water? E.g. bruises around mouth on head / arms (as if restrained)

7.03.5 Statements

- Family/next of kin – background, identification
- Medical professionals – doctors nurses psychiatric staff who can evidence any mental problem
- Any other witnesses as to circumstances, background
- Any other witnesses covering anything raised above

8

DEATHS THROUGH GUNSHOT, EXPOSURE, HEIGHTS

8.01 Deaths by Gunshot

8.01.1 Introduction

Police will always attend a death involving discharge of a firearm. Much police attention is directed towards ensuring that a death involving firearms has not been at the hands of another.

Police will be highly inclined to suspect that any death involving firearms is suspicious, and will usually require a higher degree of satisfaction before they will deem it to be "non-suspicious" and withdraw from the investigation. Many such deaths do turn out not to be "suspicious" but due to accident or suicide. The CI should attend all deaths involving firearms for reasons as outlined in Chapter 1.

8.01.2 Specific investigation guidelines – over and above the generic checklist

8.01.2.1 The deceased
- Are they the owner of the firearm?
- Do they have a licence for it?
- Are they a collector/sportsman?
- Did their occupation involve firearms use? E.g. farmer/pest control?

8.01.2.2 The finder
- Does this person own a firearm? Were they out shooting?

8.01.2.3 The body

- Are there any wounds on the body that are not consistent with known former injuries or current incident?
- Is the position consistent with the suggested sequence of events?
- Has the firearm been discharged or used in any other way?
- Is it physically possible for the deceased to have self-inflicted the wound?
- Is there an exit wound? How does it compare with the entry wound as to angle of the shot?

8.01.2.4 The scene where found

- Describe fully – indoors/outdoors
- Why was the deceased in this particular place? Familiarity/secluded/bound to be found?
- Are there other weapons at the scene?

8.01.2.5 Circumstances

- Given that this is a particularly violent death – were there any indications beforehand (if a possible suicide)
- Had something of significance recently occurred to precipitate the events?
- Was this an organised shooting event? What sort?
- Was the deceased expected to be using a firearm at that time? E.g. at work in pest control

8.01.2.6 The event

- Was the event witnessed? By whom?

8.01.2.7 Other considerations

- Is there any indication of a suicide note? Where? Is it in deceased's handwriting?
- Is there any indication of alcohol or drugs paraphernalia or tablet bottles or packets? Where?
- Is there anything unusual to suggest anything other than a suicide or an accident?

8.01.2.8 Actions

- Look for evidence to prove or disprove every possible explanation. Keep an open mind
- Take photographs
- Look for suicide note(s)
- Look for other weapons (not necessarily firearms)
- Arrange to have firearm seized by police, made safe and transported to place of safety
- Arrange to have ammunition seized by police, made safe and transported to place of safety
- Establish how many rounds have been discharged – are they all accounted for?
- Establish whether there is other ammunition inside the weapon and not yet discharged
- Are there any spent cartridges? Do the numbers tally? Do the positions tally?
- Arrange for the distance from the end of barrel to the trigger to be measured
- Arrange for the distance from fingers thumb to believed point of entry on body to be measured
- Look for other props to ensure trigger could be fired – string/rope etc; pedals in car
- If there is an exit wound on the body – look for spent casings at the scene and seize if found
- Consider arranging for testing of the firearm to ensure it could have fired any ammunition found in the body and that it actually did
- Arrange an x-ray prior to the post mortem examination to establish spread and position of bullet(s)
- Arrange toxicology

8.02 Exposure deaths

8.02.1 Introduction

Deaths through exposure are possibly rarer in England and Wales than in other countries in the world – as far as the exposure being outdoors. However they still do occur, more especially in mountainous regions. More common than exposure is hypothermia, which can happen anywhere, including indoors – more commonly in the elderly. Hypothermia differs from cold injury:

"In hypothermia the drop in core temperature may be rapid, as in immersion in near-freezing water, or slow, as in exposure to more temperate environments. The effects are proportional to the change in temperature, with metabolic rate reduced by about 10% for every 1 degree centigrade fall in temperature" *(www.patient.co.uk)*

"There may be no signs whatsoever at autopsy in a death from hypothermia and thus the history may be all-important." *(Saukko and Knight 2004)*

Cold injury is a generic term including conditions such as frost nip, frostbite and trench foot.

"Frost nip is milder than frostbite and does not usually involve tissue destruction unless it occurs repeatedly.
Frostbite involves freezing of the tissue with microvascular occlusion and subsequent tissue anoxia.
It can be graded according to its severity:

First degree: hyperaemia and oedema without skin necrosis
Second degree: large clear vesicle formation in addition to hyperaemia and oedema with partial-thickness skin necrosis
Third degree: full thickness with subcutaneous tissue necrosis, often with haemorrhagic vesicles
Fourth degree: full thickness and subcutaneous tissue necrosis, also involving muscle and bone with gangrene"
(www.patient.co.uk)

"Trench foot refer(s) to cold damp damage, whereas 'frostbite' is caused by dry conditions below zero. .. Frostbite may affect only the skin or may extend deeply into the underlying tissues." (Saukko and Knight 2004)

8.02.2 Specific investigation guidelines – over and above the generic checklist

8.02.2.1 The deceased

- Build of deceased is particularly of relevance in such cases and attention needs to be paid in this sort of death
- Previous medical conditions may have affected the person's ability to move – thus rendering them more susceptible to the hypothermia
- Previous mental incapacity may have affected the person's ability to retrieve themselves from an unusual situation – e.g. getting lost while out on a walk – thus rendering them more susceptible to the hypothermia
- Is there evidence of alcohol which speeds up the process of hypothermia
- Had they been reported as a missing person in relation to this incident?
- Had they previously gone missing and been found outdoors? If so where?

8.02.2.2 The finder

- In cases of hypothermia indoors, the status of the finder may be important – are they in a position of caring for the deceased? May there be issues of neglect to be considered?

8.02.2.3 The body

- Are there any wounds on the body that are not consistent with known former injuries or current incident?
- Is the position of the body consistent with the history given?
- What is the condition of the body
- How long has the body been there? Has it been moved after death?
- Is there any animal interference?
- Are there any body parts missing?
- Clothing – list and describe. Is it appropriate for the time of the year and the time of day?

8.02.2.4 The scene where found

- Describe fully – indoors/outdoors
- If indoors – what was the temperature? Was the heating on/not, warm/cool for the time of year?
- Outdoors - open ground/woods/beach/access routes
- Is there any indication of alcohol near the body?

8.02.2.5 Circumstances

- What were the weather conditions?
  E.g. rain/snow/freezing/fog/sunny/windy
- Area where deceased found – description
- Distance deceased found from nearest shelter of any sort – barn/house etc
- Any evidence of alcohol or drugs or medication at scene?
- Was deceased found in a shelter? Describe type/condition/heating/ventilation

8.02.2.6 The event

- The death itself is unlikely to have been witnessed (unless found alive but died in hospital) but the circumstances leading up to the disappearance will be important

8.02.2.7 The time

- If there is decomposition is there any estimation as to time of death available
- Obtain opinion from pathologist regarding stomach contents and last meal eaten

8.02.2.8 Actions

- Photographs of the scene where found if outdoors will be very helpful for the Coroner's inquest
- Provide a map showing where the deceased lived, stayed and where found with the route highlighted

8.02.2.9 Additional statements

- A report should be obtained from the senior police office in charge of any search effort if one was made

8.03 Deaths and heights

The discovery and initial investigation of such deaths will depend somewhat on whether the body is at ground level, the deceased having descended from above (e.g. a multi-storey building or car park); or whether the deceased is at the foot of cliffs (e.g. on the coast or in a quarry where the ground level as such is above the deceased). Thereafter the enquiries are much the same for both locations.

8.03.1 The deceased

- Past visits to this location?
- Previous knowledge of the place as a good spot to die?
- What is the person wearing? Day/night/any clothing?
- Medical/psychiatric history?

8.03.2 The finder

- Was this person known to the deceased – were they together?
- What was this person doing to be there and find the deceased/see the event?
- Were there other people in the group who saw what happened and can reassure that the finder is not implicated?
- Is this person a regular body finder?

8.03.3 The body

- Check there are no injuries on the body that might indicate a struggle prior to the "fall" – e.g. restraint marks on hands and feet; tape/gag marks around mouth; puncture wounds

8.03.4 The scene if a cliff top or quarry top

- Why did this person come to this place to jump?
- Did they leave anything to draw attention to their action?

- Cliffs? Obtain information as to the height from coastguard or recovery team. This will be relevant to the Coroner and the family may want to know
- Location – if cliffs establish grid reference from coastguard or helicopter etc

8.03.5 The scene if at ground level e.g. from a building

- Why did this person come to this place to jump? Did they live/stay/work there?
- Where is the starting point? How is this known?
- How did they get to the starting point? Lift/stairs? Were these accessible? Should they have been?
- Building – try and estimate – how many floors – average height per floor
- Is the building public / private / housing / office / other?

8.03.6 The event

- Was the event witnessed? By whom?

8.03.7 Other considerations

- Is there any indication of a suicide note? Where? Is it in deceased's handwriting?
- Ask the recovery team (if applicable) to look for other items close to the body
- Notoriety of this location for deaths by suicide or accident?
- Is there any indication of alcohol or drugs paraphernalia or tablet bottles or packets? Where?
- Was there a party prior?
- Is there CCTV coverage of the location?
- Is there anything unusual to suggest anything other than a suicide or an accident?

8.03.8 Actions if a cliff top or quarry top

- Look for suicide note(s)
- Take photographs of "top scene" and "bottom scene"
- Request any CCTV tapes where available

- Consider identification methods – is visual possible? If not – is dental available
- Arrange toxicology for drugs and alcohol

8.03.9 Alternative actions if at ground level e.g. from a building

- Take photographs of "top scene" and "bottom scene"
- Check there are no signs of forced entry to relevant area of building
- Check there are no signs of struggle in relevant area of building
- Check there is no evidence of chloroform or other stupefying agents (possibly used to render person insensible prior to being pushed out of window with no struggle)
- Measure the opening of the window/door, the height of the window ledge from the floor of the room within
- Is there a window opening limiter? Does it appear faulty? Similarly for window catches
- Check for signs of damage on the window sill (possible evidence of being forced through the aperture) – or absence of such signs
- Look for evidence of tablets or drugs / alcohol containers
- Look for suicide note(s)
- Request any CCTV tapes where available
- Consider identification methods. Is visual possible? If not – is dental available?
- Arrange toxicology for drugs and alcohol

8.03.10 Additional statements

- Coastguard or body recovery team if relevant
- Witnesses to the event itself (may well be strangers if at a beauty spot)
- Premises/building owner/manager may be appropriate – including how access was gained and whether lawful or not
- Family/carers as well as usual information e.g. identification, social history, background, past suicidal ideation/attempts to specifically include any past incidents involving heights/visits to this location

8.03.11 Marine and Coastguard Agency (MCA) and Her Majesty's Coastguard (HMCG)

The Coastguard Agency is a very helpful resource in asisisting with the recovery of bodies from geographically awkward locations. This is not only when the coastline is involved but also applies for other locations such as quarries. On the search and rescue (SAR) page of the MCA website it states:

"The Maritime and Coastguard Agency (MCA) provides a response and co-ordination service for maritime SAR.... The SAR role is undertaken by HM Coastguard, which is responsible for the initiation and co-ordination of civil maritime SAR. This includes the mobilisation, organisation and tasking of adequate resources to respond to persons either in distress at sea, or on those inland waters listed in paragraph 4.2, or to persons at risk of injury or death on the cliffs and shoreline of the UK. As part of its response, HM Coastguard provides Coastguard Rescue Teams for cliff and shoreline search and rescue purposes."
www.mcga.gov.uk

See chapter 3 for further on the role of the Maritime and Coastguard Agency.

9

DEATHS IN HEALTHCARE SETTINGS

9.01 Introduction

Deaths in healthcare settings will usually be initially reported to the ME via the MEO who will have a working relationship with the GPs, hospital and hospice doctors in that jurisdiction. See Chapter 1 for more information on the proposed death certification process as contained in the Coroners and Justice Bill and in the DH programme overview paper 2008 on the process of death certification (op cit).

Deaths will be referred to the MEOs by GPs daily. A small percentage of such referrals will have occurred actually in the surgery itself, or within a short time after the patient has been to the surgery. The fact that there may be a working relationship between the MEO and the GP should not numb the MEO to the possibility of something more untoward having occurred. There are occasions where an individual or group of individuals within the medical profession may abuse their position of trust and commit deliberate acts of homicide. When the MEO suspects that something like this has occurred they will advise the ME who will refer the death through to the Coroner.

There will be occasions when it is obvious that a death will need immediate referral to the Coroner and the CI will start the investigations from the beginning. On some occasions a death in a healthcare setting may be referred directly to the police or to the Coroner.

9.02 The CI

As discussed in Chapter 1 the CI needs to have good medical knowledge. They will also need a good understanding of the organisation involved in any particular death and the possible aspects of the death that will need to be investigated.

The investigation of deaths that occur in healthcare settings and care environments can prove different and sometimes challenging difficult for CIs.

CIs will need their usual sensitivity when dealing with health care professionals that they use in the investigation of any death. At the same time the CI needs to conduct a thorough, impartial and rigorous investigation.

9.03 Records

The CI will need to know what records and in particular what medical records are available that should be obtained as part of their investigations on behalf of the Coroner, and how to obtain those records. The Shipman Inquiry Report (2003) commented:

"Even if the autopsy is taking place in the hospital where the deceased died, the medical records are not always examined. Some coroners and their officers provide high quality information for pathologists and are prepared to make any further enquiries requested. However, others are less efficient. Coroner's officers may be office-bound, may have no investigative role and may be unable to identify or discover further information which could be of assistance to the pathologist." (op cit para 9.20)

If the organisation concerned does not want to release the records that the Coroner requires a new power has become available to Coroners in the Coroners and Justice Bill:

The Senior Coroner.... if authorised in writing by the Chief Coroner.... may enter and search any land specified in the authorisation. Schedule 4 Paragraph 3(1)

So long as certain conditions are satisfied: Schedule 4 Paragraph 3(2) and 3(3) (op cit)

Schedule 4 Paragraph 3(4) states

"Where the senior coroner is lawfully on any land, he may
a) seize anything which is on the land, and
b) inspect and take copies of any documents"

9.04 Outcomes

9.04.1 Inquest hearing

A death may be considered an expected outcome of the individual's illness or a reflection of the very real risk associated with some medical conditions and their treatment. In some circumstances a Coroner may decide to have an investigative inquest into the matter, in others the Coroner may decide not to. Even if there is to be an inquest hearing, a verdict of death by natural causes may be returned at the end of the inquest hearing after examination of all the facts.

The evidence may indicate that the death was a result of what could be described as an "adverse clinical event". This could be as a result of an equipment failure, or of a unintended error by a health care professional. It is hard to imagine that a Coroner would not order an inquest in circumstances such as these.

9.04.2 Civil suit

There is a possibility that an individual may have been involved in an unintended "human factors error", in which case civil suit may arise at some stage.

9.04.3 Corporate Manslaughter

If the evidence indicates that the death was a result of an "adverse clinical event" due to an inappropriate system of working, then the Corporate Manslaughter and Corporate Homicide Act 2007 may be relevant.

Section 1 of the Act defines the offence:

(1) An organisation to which this section applies is guilty of an offence if the way in which its activities are managed or organised—
(a) causes a person's death, and
(b) amounts to a gross breach of a relevant duty of care owed by the organisation to the deceased.

9.04.4 Homicide

Another possibility to consider is that of a "mercy killing" by a relative or even by a member of staff. This may amount to a deliberate act of homicide when defined as "hastening death".

Under circumstances such as these latter two, then the police do become involved then liaison will need to take place as described at sections 1.15.2 and 1.15.3 above. See also the MOU: "Investigating patient safety incidents (unexpected death of serious untoward harm): a protocol for liaison and effective communications between the National Health Service, Association of Chief Police Officers and Health & Safety Executive" (2006), which is available to download from the DH website www.dh.gov.uk.

If there is sufficient evidence for the Crown Prosecution Service (CPS) to prosecute for any such offence then there may not be a need for a Coroner to have a full inquest hearing as the matter could be adjourned under section 16 of the Coroners Act 1988. In the Coroners and Justice Bill the adjournment is referred to as "suspension" under Chapter 1 section 14 and Schedule 1 Part 1.

9.05 Regulatory organisations

9.05.1 Care Quality Commission (CQC)

The Care Quality Commission (CQC) was established under the Health and Social Care Act 2008 and came into existence on 1st October 2008.

From 1st April 2009 the CQC replaced the Commission for Social Care Inspection (CSCI), the Healthcare Commission and the Mental Health Act Commission (MHAC).

The CQC website stated in July 2009:

"The Care Quality Commission is the independent regulator of health and social care in England. Our aim is to make sure better care is provided for everyone, whether that's in hospital, in care homes, in people's own homes, or elsewhere. We regulate health and adult social care services, whether provided by the NHS, local authorities, private companies or voluntary organisations." www.cqc.org.uk

The rationale for a new organisation to replace the preceding three was stated on the CQC website in February 2009:

As the needs of people who use social care and health services, carers and their families have changed over the last decade, responsibility for social care and health services has come together.... Now the Care Quality Commisisons will be the first opportunity to brign these functions together under one iundependent regulator." www.cqc.org.uk

As the CQC website is dynamic, with its contents changing as the role and parameters of the Commission become clearer, every CI should visit the website www.cqc.org.uk regularly and download the assorted documents available.

The new system is meant to enable a joined up regulation for health and social care, helping to ensure better outcomes for the people who use services.

Health and social care providers - including, for the first time, NHS providers - are required to register with the new regulator in order to provide services.

The Act gave the Commission a wider range of enforcement powers along with flexibility on how and when to use them. This allows the regulator greater powers to achieve compliance with registration requirements - including requirements relating to infection control. The Commission is able to apply specific conditions to respond to specific risks - such as requiring a ward or service to be closed until safety requirements met, as well as being able to suspend or de-register services where absolutely necessary.

Of particular relevance to Coroners and CIs is a 2008 guidance document on healthcare associated infection (HCAI): Registering with the Care Quality Commission in relation to healthcare associated infection: Guidance for trusts 2009/10. This is available to download as a pdf from the CQC website www.cqc.gov.uk. It states that there will be:

"new legal requirements on trusts to protect patients and staff from healthcare associated infections (HCAI)" (op cit)

These requirements came into force from 1 April 2009 and will:

"apply to all healthcare services that are provided by the following NHS trusts in 2008/09:
• Acute trusts (both foundation and non-foundation trusts)
• Ambulance trusts
• Mental health trusts (including learning disability trusts)
• Primary care trusts
• NHS Blood and Transplant
They do not currently apply to commissioners or commissioned services (such as dental practices and GP surgeries), independent healthcare or social care. However, plans for regulation of other types of care providers are being developed in 2009. (op cit July 2009)

It is possible to see the CQC assessment of any service provider on the CQC website.

9.05.2 National Patient Safety Agency (NPSA)

The NPSA is described on its website as:

"The National Patient Safety Agency leads and contributes to improved, safe patient care by informing, supporting and influencing the health sector. We are an Arm's Length Body of the Department of Health and are responsible for helping improve patient care." www.npsa.nhs.uk

There are three divisions: the Patient Safety Division, the National Clinical Assessment Service and the National Research Ethics Service. The functions of these three divisions is explained in more detail in their leaflet which is available on their website: www.npsa.nhs.uk

The NPSA commissions and monitors three national Confidential Enquiries into Suicide and Homicide by People with Mental Illness; Maternal and Child Health; and Patient Outcome and Death.

There is a leaflet available from their website to download (English and Welsh versions) in which they explain that they pay for and monitor:

"suicide and homicide by people with mental illness (suicide or murder by people who have been cared for by mental health services);
• maternal and child health (improving the health of mothers, babies and children); and
• patient outcome and death (how and whether patients recover following healthcare treatment)"

The NPSA run a National Reporting and Learning System (NRLS) and the relevant page on the NPSA website states:

"Patient safety is our priority. We aim to improve patient care with rapid responses to incidents, analysis of incidents that come to us via the National Reporting and Learning System and the collaborative development of actions that can be implemented locally." (www.npsa.nhs.uk/nrls)

It further states:

"Although each event is unique, there are likely to be similarities and patterns which and will go unnoticed if they are not reported. All NHS organisations can learn from what has happened in one service without other patients being put at risk." (www.npsa.nhs.uk/nrls)

Coroners are not obliged to advise the NPSA of any unintended or unexpected incident during the provision of healthcare which may have led to the death of a patient, but some may choose to do so.

9.05.2.1 'Never events'

As mentioned at section 6.04.4 above there is a 2009 NPSA NRLS document about the never events framework 2009/10. This document is available from the NPSA NRLS website (www.npsa.nhs.uk/nrls) to download in pdf format. The framework identifies an initial core list of eight "never events" which are defined as:

"serious, largely preventable patient safety incidents that should not occur if the available preventative measures have been implemented".

See also sections 6.04.3.11 above and 10.2, 10.3, 11.02.6, 11.03.7, 11.04.2, 12.02.5 below for more about 'never events'.

9.05.3 National Clinical Assessment Service (NCAS)

The NCAS is a division of the NPSA and came into existence in April 2005 following the National Clinical Assessment Authority (Establishment and Constitution) Amendment Order 2004

The NCAS includes within its remit doctors' performance, salaried dentists and dentists in general practice and will include pharmacists from April 2009

Visit www.ncas.npsa.nhs.uk

9.05.4 Professional bodies

There are also regulatory bodies such as the General Medical Council (GMC) in respect of doctors, the General Dental Council (GDC) and the Nursing and Midwifery Council (NMC). These exist to set and enforce professional standards and conduct in respect of relevant professionals.

Visit www.gmc-uk.org; www.gdc-uk.org and www.nmc-uk.org for more information on the roles of these three professional bodies.

9.05.5 Medicines and Healthcare products Regulatory Agency (MHRA)

If medical equipment or medication is involved in the death then the MHRA should be consulted. They have a responsibility to ensure the safety of medical equipment and medicines.

On the front page of their website www.mhra.gov.uk it states that the MHRA is:

"the government agency which is responsible for ensuring that medicines and medical devices work, and are acceptably safe.
• We keep watch over medicines and devices, and we take any necessary action to protect the public promptly if there is a problem.
• We aim to make as much information as possible publicly available.
• We encourage everyone - the public and healthcare professionals as well as industry - to tell us about any problems with a medicine or medical device, so that we can investigate and take any necessary action. "

There is a 2008 document entitled "Medicines and Medical Devices Regulation: What you need to know" and this is available to download in pdf format from the MHRA wesbite. This document discusses the licensing of medicines and the authorisation of medical devices.

9.05.5.1 Herbal remedies

The MHRA also considers herbal remedies to some extent and

"is working with herbal practitioners and the government to introduce safeguards for this type of treatment. Details of any herbal product found to contain potentially harmful ingredients, or which interacts with conventional medicines, are posted on the MHRA website. The Agency has also recently introduced a new scheme for regulating homeopathic remedies." www.mhra.gov.uk

9.05.5.2 MHRA Recalls and alerts

"When a product is suspected or known to be faulty, the MHRA immediately works with manufacturers and wholesalers on the most appropriate and timely action to take."

"Warnings (Alerts) can be issued about defective medicines, problems with devices, and side effects associated with medicines and blood and blood products. These are sent out to healthcare professionals and organisations, and publicised widely in print and online, including on the MHRA website."

"The MHRA's Defective Medicines Report Centre (DMRC) issues alerts to healthcare professionals, hospitals, GP surgeries, and wholesalers to tell them when a medicine is being recalled or when there are concerns about the quality that will affect its safety or effectiveness." www.mhra.gov.uk

Coroners and CIs can ask to be on the email circulation list about queries over medicines. They can also check to see if a warning was issued where there is any suspicion about any medicine taken. The MHRA can conduct examinations of medical equipment and give opinions as to operation and defects.

9.05.6 Health and Safety Executive (HSE)

Most Coroners do not consider that deaths in local general hospitals will need to involve the Health and Safety Executive even though the location of such deaths will in most instances involve a "workplace environment". However there is a protocol for liaison between HSE and the police "Work-Related Deaths: A Protocol for liaison" (2003) between the HSE and police that

Coroners will consider. This is available to download from the HSE website: www.hse.gov.uk.

Additionally from November 2007 there is a Memorandum of Understanding, to be reviewed annually, between the Coroner Society of England and Wales (CSEW) and the HSE available to download from the HSE website, which states it :

"is intended to promote and continue effective working relationships between Coroners and HM Inspectors of Health and Safety, with the object of fostering constructive co-operation." (op cit)

In any case where HSE could possibly "have an interest" they should be contacted at an early stage.
One of the stated aims of the MOU is:

"To set out clearly the level of assistance that HSE can legitimately provide to the Coroner following a work-related death." (op cit)

The HSE may have specialist expertise which will help the Coroner and thus the CI in identifying the normal working practices in the establishment, and in eliciting what happened in a particular instance.

The HSE may need to consider prosecution in some instances.

CIs may encounter a dilemma in investigating cases where the HSE are involved. This is around how much separate (and independent) investigation they do or arrange on behalf of their Coroner. There is an understandable reluctance to duplicate enquiries. However, there is the potential for compromising the Coroner's investigation if a separate investigation is not carried out.

It is possible that avenues of enquiry might not be pursued if the investigation is left entirely to the HSE, as their focus is necessarily different. The HSE focus is around whether any prosecution should follow. Moreover disclosure to the Coroner from HSE can be accompanied by a request for an undertaking not to use such evidence at the inquest hearing for fear it may have an adverse effect on any prosecution.

The MOU attempts to address this:

"The Coroner alone is responsible for deciding on the scope or ambit of the inquest. The Coroner must ensure that the relevant facts are fully and fairly investigated and are the subject of public scrutiny during the inquest hearing. The wider public interest also includes the need to ensure that the risk of prejudice to any ongoing investigation and potential criminal proceedings is minimised." (op cit)
The front page of the HSE website states:

"HSE's job is to protect people against risks to health or safety arising out of work activities. "Our mission is to protect people's health and safety by ensuring risks in the changing workplace are properly controlled."
We do this through research, information and advice, promoting training, new or revised regulations and codes of practice, inspection, investigation and enforcement" (www.hse.gov.uk)

Visit their website www.hse.gov.uk for other useful information.

The government's position paper (2004) states:

"Coroners could provide an additional safeguard by having a power to conduct **targeted further investigations**, *(sic) as suggested by the Fundamental Review and the Shipman Inquiry .... Effectiveness would be enhanced if lines of responsibility were strengthened between the coroner and other investigating agencies, such as the Health and Safety Executive."* (op cit paragraph 43)

In addition, as mentioned above, a Memorandum of Understanding between the NHS, ACPO and the HSE about investigating patient safety incidents was formalised in February 2006. Visit www.dh.gov.uk to download a pdf format of this document. The protocol is intended to help the three agencies:

"• meet their responsibilities for the safety of patients and NHS staff
• make clear to one another from the outset their particular statutory responsibilities
• set out their own operational needs
• prompt early decisions about the actions and investigation(s) thought to be necessary by all organisations and a dialogue about the implications of these
• provide an efficient and effective approach to the management of the investigation(s)
• develop and strengthen partnership working
• prompt the identification of lead personnel to manage liaison between the three agencies
• save time and other resources of all the agencies concerned" (op cit)

9.06 Guidance

9.06.1 National Institute for Health and Clinical Excellence (NICE)

Coroners and their Investigators would also benefit from an awareness of NICE. There is a document entitled "NICE: our guidance sets the standard for good healthcare" which is available in pdf format to download from their website: www.nice.org.uk. This outlines the format of NICE, what it does and how it works. The front page of the NICE website states:

"NICE is an independent organisation responsible for providing national guidance on promoting good health and preventing and treating ill health.

NICE produces guidance in three areas of health:
• public health - guidance on the promotion of good health and the prevention of ill health for those working in the NHS, local authorities and the wider public and voluntary sector
• health technologies - guidance on the use of new and existing medicines, treatments and procedures within the NHS
• clinical practice - guidance on the appropriate" (www.nice.org.uk)

The guidelines NICE have already produced and have in development may prove to be useful to Coroners and CIs in their understanding of the treatment and criteria for treatment of certain illnesses.

Guidelines exist on many conditions that can result in the death of a patient and which should therefore be provided to the Coroner in any case where there is to be an inquest hearing. Guidelines are available both for professionals and for members of the public (including therefore patients themselves). For example there are guidelines on: management of head injury; management of atrial fibrillation; pressure ulcer management; prevention of falls in older people; prevention of healthcare-associated infections in primary and community care; management and prevention of self-harm.

There are many other NICE guideline papers and there is a comprehensive index on the website listing completed guidelines and those being developed. Even where a guidance document has not yet been finalised it is possible to print off the draft proposal and scope document which would assist the Coroner at an inquest hearing.

9.07 Experts

The Coroner can consider the use of experts to assist in the inquest process. Such experts might include: senior nurse; surgeon; physician; anaesthetist etc.

9.07.1 ECRI Institute (ECRI)

ECRI (originally established as the Emergency Care Research Institute) is an independent health services research agency employing over 280 people internationally.

Its website states:

"ECRI Institute, a not for profit organisation, dedicates itself to bringing the discipline of applied scientific research in healthcare to uncover the best approaches to improving patient care. As pioneers in this science for 40 years, ECRI Institute marries experience and independence with the objectivity of evidence-based research.

More than 5,000 healthcare organisations worldwide rely on ECRI Institute's expertise in patient safety improvement, risk and quality management, healthcare processes, devices, procedures, and drug technology.

ECRI Institute is a totally independent non profit research agency and a Collaborating Centre of the World Health Organisation for Patient Safety, Risk Management and Health Care Technology.

All of ECRI Institute's products and services are available through the European Office, but at the same time addressing the special requirements of the region. For example, consulting services to the NHS, accident and forensic investigations, conferences, exhibitions, reports, research, are all carried out and organised by our UK staff. Utilising some of the world's largest health related databases, assistance, support and guidance can be given to our UK and European clients at local level."
(www.ecri.org.uk/about-ecri.htm)

ECRI Institute provides investigative support reviewing clinical practice or procedures in serious healthcare incidents including provision of strategic advice to SIOs in cases where gross negligence or corporate homicide is suspected in hospital, care home or community settings. They also provide expert advice and examination in relation to incidents involving medical devices and implants when such devices may be suspected as being a contributory factor. Visit the website at www.ecri.org.uk.

The Shipman Inquiry Report (2003) comments in cases where there may have been medical error or neglect:

"Such investigations should not be undertaken by the police unless there is a suspicion of criminality. If the investigation discovered facts suggesting that there had been neglect or error serious enough to warrant the consideration of criminal proceedings, the coroner could always refer the case to the police at that stage ... Death investigations in which any issue of medical error or neglect arises require particular expertise. I shall suggest that, if there is any degree of complexity, such investigations should be conducted by a specialist team of investigators." (op cit 9.74)

9.07.2 Specialists

The Shipman Inquiry comments significantly for CIs that there should be:

"A small team of "coroner's investigators" at every regional office who can develop expertise in medical cases." (op cit Ch 19 and recommendations 34 – 36)

It is vital that any CI investigating a death in a medical institution has medical knowledge or has received adequate training. Such knowledge should include:

- Anatomy
- Physiology
- Drugs - their names, spellings, uses, effects and side effects
- Medical abbreviations
- An ability to navigate notes and records
- Hierarchies of staff
- Systems within the organisation concerned

Thomas et al (2002) pages 35 ff consider hospital deaths. The book looks at matters from a legal practitioner's perspective. CIs can best assist their Coroner if they have anticipated all likely questions the practitioner and the family may ask at inquest – so long as it is relevant to the four questions relating to the death: "who, where, when and how". If questions raised are not relevant to those four areas then the Coroner should not be concerned with them unless Article 2 of the European Convention on Human Rights issues is being considered (see section 6.01.6 for more about Article 2 investigations).

9.08 Potential difficulties

9.08.1 Families' expectations

There may be some dissatisfaction on behalf of a deceased's family in relation to the care of patients within health care institutions. There may be other cases where the family did not have a concern, but the Coroner's investigations uncover issues of concern to the Coroner.

No matter how the concern arose, families have expectations of the inquest process that are not always accurate. There is a need for CIs to provide appropriate support to family members but at the same time ensure that their expectations regarding any Coroner's inquest hearing are not unrealistic in terms of the answers it can provide.

An explanation of the purposes of the inquest as set out in rule 36 of the Coroners Rules 1984, and of the limitations of the inquest process can be helpful. It needs supplementing with an explanation to the family of their ability to raise concerns with the organisation concerned, independent of the inquest.

"(1) The proceedings and evidence at an inquest shall be directed solely to ascertaining the following matters, namely:-

(a) who the deceased was

(b) how, when and where the deceased came by his death

(c) the particulars for the time being required by the Registration Acts to be registered concerning the death

(2) Neither the coroner nor the jury shall express any opinion on any other matters" (Coroners Rules 1984 Rule 36)

The purposes of the "investigation" as it is termed in the Coroners and Justice Bill, as opposed to "inquest" are set out in paragraph 5:

"The purpose of an investigation under this Part into a person's death is to ascertain—

(a) who the deceased was;

(b) how, when and where the deceased came by his or her death;

(c) the particulars (if any) required by the 1953 Act to be registered concerning the death."

Suggestions as to use of the Patient Advisory Liaison Service (PALS) system and of their ability to take legal advice may also help.

The PALS website www.pals.nhs.uk states:

*"The **Patient Advice and Liaison Service**, (sic) known as PALS, has been introduced to ensure that the NHS listens to patients, their relatives, carers and friends, and answers their questions and resolves their concerns as quickly as possible.*

In particular PALS will

• Provide you with information about the NHS and help you with any other health-related enquiry

• Help resolve concerns or problems when you are using the NHS

• Provide information about the NHS complaints procedure and how to get independent help if you decide you may want to make a complaint

Visit www.pals.nhs.uk for more information about PALS. Additionally many local PALS have their own websites which can be accessed through the main website.

9.08.1.1 Independent Complaints Advocacy Service (ICAS)

ICAS is a free service available since 2003 and delivered by four voluntary sector organisations: Citizen's Advice Bureaux (CAB); the Carers Federation; POhWER; and South East Advocacy Projects (SEAP). It is run on a regional basis.

It provides support to people in England wishing to complain about the treatment or care they received under the National Health Service (NHS).

It assists with complaints about GPs, Dentists, Ambulance services, Hospitals. It offers experienced advocates and caseworkers to help make a complaint. More details about ICAS can be found on the Department of Health website www.dh.gov.uk and also at www.adviceguide.org.uk and follow the links through Your Family then Health.

9.08.1.2 NHS Litigation Authority (NHSLA)

The NHSLA was established in 1995 under section 11 of the National Health Service and Community Care Act 1990. According to information from its website, www.nhsla.com, it is a Special Health Authority (part of the NHS), responsible for handling negligence claims made against NHS bodies in England. In addition to dealing with claims when they arise, it has an active risk management programme to help raise standards of care in the NHS and hence reduce the number of incidents leading to claims. It also monitors human rights case-law on behalf of the NHS through a Human Rights Act Information Service. It publishes an annual report and a series of "fact sheets".

There is a section on the NHSLA website entitled "Advice for Clinicians" which states:-

WHAT DOES THE PATIENT NEED TO PROVE?
- *that the treatment fell below a minimum standard of competence; and*
- *that he/she has suffered an injury; and*
- *that it is more likely than not that the injury would have been avoided, or less severe, with proper treatment.*

WHAT IS THE TIME LIMIT FOR MAKING A CLAIM?
The basic rule is three years from the date of injury, but it can be longer if:
- *the patient is a child, when the three year period only begins on his/her eighteenth birthday.*
- *the patient has a mental disorder within the meaning of the Mental Health Act 1983 so as to be incapable of managing his/her own affairs, when the three year period is suspended.*
- *there was an interval before the patient realised or could reasonably have found out that he/she had suffered a significant injury possibly related to his/her treatment.*
- *a court is persuaded that it is fair overall to allow a longer period.*

There is also a section entitled: Info for Patients in which members of public are encouraged to seek legal advice and to consult with the organisation Action against Medical Accidents (AvMA).

9.08.1.3 Action against Medical Accidents (AvMA)

The front page of their website states:

"Action against Medical Accidents (AvMA) is the independent charity which promotes better patient safety and justice for people who have been affected by a medical accident. A 'medical accident' is where avoidable harm has been caused as a result of treatment or failure to treat appropriately. AvMA believes that whatever the cause of a medical accident, the people affected deserve explanations, support, and where appropriate, compensation. Furthermore, we all deserve to know that the necessary steps will be taken to prevent similar accidents being repeated.

We provide free and confidential advice and support to people affected by medical accidents, via our helpline and casework service and can refer to our panel of specialist clinical negligence solicitors or other sources of support where appropriate." (www.avma.org.uk)

9.08.2 Staff concerns

It is not often the case that the cause of death in a medical institution is attributable to only one factor.   For example many surgical operations and interventions have known risks. Some surgeons and physicians are more prepare than others to treat a particular patient where the risk factors are higher.

The CQC assesses one Trust against another and this information is available on the website may be relevant for the Coroner at an inquest hearing.

The Coroner may want to ask questions of the doctor as to the known risks of a procedure or treatment; as to any correlation between other factors for that patient; as to drug interactions, for example. It is the task of the CI to ensure as much of that information is available to the Coroner in advance of the hearing itself.

In other cases the patient themselves may have additional risk factor(s) / pre-morbidities / co-pathologies. It is possible that even in the hands of a professional carrying out their role carefully and skilfully, the outcome of any treatment may result in the death of an individual.

Similarly, there are other occasions where medical negligence may be a contributory factor towards the cause of death (see above). However, often the evidence available falls short of this but nevertheless should be drawn to the attention of other bodies within the medical profession in order that action against individuals or specific institutions may follow.

Healthcare professionals may fear that they could face disciplinary action and may want to refer to their professional body or medical defence organisation upon becoming aware of a Coroner's investigation before agreeing to speak to a CI.

9.08.3 The organisation

The organisation itself may be concerned about possibilities of criminal or civil prosecution and may want to refer to their legal advisers upon becoming aware of a Coroner's investigation before agreeing to speak to a CI.

At a talk to the COA on 10/7/2008 in Nottingham, two different solicitors (one of whom is a Deputy Coroner) spoke about the fact that in some cases the Trust will have their own legal team, while an individual member of staff will have their own (different) legal representation.

In such circumstances, the Coroner and the CI will need to liaise with both teams of lawyers.

Lawyers will often have their own statements taken from their client. The CI needs to alert the Coroner to any such scenario so that issues of disclosure can be resolved in advance of a hearing itself. The value of a Pre-Inquest Review (PIR) cannot be over-emphasised, even though it has no status in law.

The Department of Health issued a document in October 2005 entitled: "When a Patient Dies: Advice on Developing Bereavement Services in the NHS". This is available to download in pdf format from the Department of Health website www.dh.gov.uk and contains useful information for Coroners and CIs.

10

DEATHS IN PRIMARY HEALTHCARE SETTINGS

10.01 Introduction

This chapter concentrates on aspects specifically relevant to deaths in primary healthcare settings and should be read in conjunction with Chapter 9 which is generic for all deaths in healthcare settings and in conjunction with Chapter 1.

Deaths in primary care include deaths which arise from doctors' surgeries and more rarely dental surgeries as well as deaths within the care of the ambulance service.

10.02 Deaths in doctors' surgeries

These deaths will usually be reported straight to the ME office and may be dealt with entirely within the ME system. See Chapter 1 for more information on the proposed death certification process as contained in the Coroners and Justice Bill and in the DH programme overview paper 2008 on the process of death certification (op cit). However if there is any concern, either from the patient's family, or from the ME, the death will be referred on to the Coroner.

If the ME system deals with such a death, then in all likelihood the doctor will issue the MCCD in the usual way and the ME, having scrutinised and satisfied himself, will complete the process and there will not need to be a post mortem examination. This is because patients with existing illnesses may die in any location and just because it occurs within the doctor's surgery does not necessarily make the death "suspicious" or untoward.

Indeed some might argue that as the patient has just seen the doctor (in some instances) the circumstances of issuing the MCCD may be totally satisfied.

However there will be occasions when such a death raises cause for concern.

10.02.1 Family concerns

The family may be dissatisfied with the treatment that the deceased had been receiving from the doctor and make their concerns known. Those concerns may or may not be justifiable and the CMI / MEO will make initial enquiries as to the grounds for the concerns.

If the concerns are judged to be reasonable by the ME, then the death will be referred to the Coroner and a post mortem examination will take place.

The results may then allay the family's concerns. They may show that the doctor's professional judgment and treatment of the patient was accurate. They may show that there was an underlying illness or disease of which the doctor was unaware.

The Shipman Inquiry Report (2003) stated

"The aim of the Coroner Service should be to provide an independent, cohesive system of death investigation and certification, readily accessible to and understood by the public. For every death, it should seek to identify the deceased, to discover where, how and why the deceased died and should provide an explanation for the death to those associated with the deceased or having a proper interest in understanding the cause and circumstances of the death." (op cit para 19.13)

10.02.2 Doctors' concerns

The doctor may have seen the patient but not been able to establish the illness or disease from which the patient was suffering and have planned to arrange further tests or further referrals.

The doctor may state that although they had just seen the patient the existing co-pathologies were so complex and many, that they do not know which caused the death.

The doctor may have just carried out a procedure, including surgery, or administered new or stronger medication.

In such circumstances as these (a non-exhaustive sample) the doctor is unlikely to wish to issue an MCCD, and even if they did so issue, it would be unlikely to be acceptable to the ME and thence to the Coroner.

10.02.3 Had not seen the doctor

The doctor may not have seen the patient – who may have died in the waiting room. It may be that an appointment had been kept with another health practitioner, e.g. a nurse, therapist, dietician etc. In such circumstances, unless the doctor had previously seen the patient within the required time period and be able to issue the MCCD, one would not be forthcoming.

10.02.4 Specific investigation guidelines for an inquest – over and above the generic checklist

10.02.4.1 Circumstances

- What had the patient been doing in the surgery?
- Had there been any procedure or surgery?
  If so describe fully; had the doctor performed this procedure/surgery before? Were there any unexpected events during the procedure/surgery?
- What is the usual risk level involved in this sort of procedure/surgery? Was it raised for any reason? E.g. the pre-existing condition of the patient?
- Is it possible that there has been an adverse reaction to any anaesthetic? If so full details of the anaesthetic drugs, amounts and their effects will be needed
- Did the deceased have any previously diagnosed diseases injuries or illnesses that would have knowingly increased the risk of this procedure? E.g. was there a pre-existing cardiac condition? Was the patient on Warfarin or other anti-thrombolytic drugs?

- Were there additional complications found during the procedure/surgery that were previously unforeseen?
- Was the procedure/surgery elective or emergency?
- Were there any previously known allergies?
- Had the patient seen another health practitioner? If so why?
- What did that other practitioner do? Eg take a blood sample? Perform massage/osteopathy/reflexology?

10.02.4.2 Actions

- Seize any potential evidence – e.g. equipment / drugs
- Take photographs of equipment before moved (if possible)
- Seize any medical notes & photocopy them immediately

10.02.4.3 Statements

The existing working relationship that the CIs will have with the doctors and their surgery staff may help facilitate access to all necessary areas.

As each individual case varies so will the witnesses from whom statements will be needed. They may include (but may not be limited to) any of the following:

- Doctor who performed procedure / surgery
- Any other staff member who was present
- Any other health practitioner who was with the patient

10.02.5 'Never events' and doctors' surgeries

Events one, two, four and eight on the core list of 'never events' would apply if the 'event' had occurred at a doctors' surgery (see section 9.05.2.1 above):

Event one on the core list refers to 'wrong site surgery' which is described as:

"A surgical intervention performed on the wrong site (for example wrong knee, wrong eye, wrong patient, wrong limb, or wrong organ); the incident is detected after the operation and the patient requires further surgery, on the correct site, and/or may have complications following the wrong surgery." (op cit)

It specifically relates to:

"Organisations that provide major, minor and/or day case surgery."

Appendix A of the framework document states:

"Operating on the wrong site can have devastating consequences for patients."
(op cit)

Appendix A advises implementation of guidance from the World Health Organisation and the use of a surgical safety checklist to prevent wrong site surgery.
See www.npsa.nhs.uk/nrls/alerts-and-directives/alerts/safer-surgery-alert

It also advises use of standard wristbands to reduce the possibility of the wrong patient receiving the surgery.
See www.npsa.nhs.uk/nrls/alerts-and-directives/notices/wristbands

Event two on the core list refers to 'retained instrument post-operation' which is described as:

"One or more instruments are unintentionally retained following an operative procedure, and an operation or other invasive procedure is needed to remove this, and/or there are complications to the patient arising from its continued presence. This Never Event does not include interventional radiology or cardiology procedures, and the definition of instrument does not include guide wires, screws, swabs or other similar material." *(op cit)*

It specifically relates to:

"Organisations that provide major, minor and/or day case surgery."

Appendix A of the framework document states:

"Unintentionally retained instruments are a potential cause of complications and repeat surgery. Most providers will have developed their own local policies based on available advice."

Appendix A refers to various advice documents which CIs can access if the need arises.

Event four on the core list refers to 'misplaced naso or orogastric tube not detected prior to use' which is described as:

"Naso or orogastric tube placed in the respiratory tract rather than the gastrointestinal tract and not detected prior to commencing feeding or other use.." (op cit)

It relates to:

"All care settings."

Appendix A of the framework document states:

"There is a risk that nasogastric or orogastric feeding tubes may be inserted in a lung or bronchus instead of the stomach, resulting in potentially serious harm and/or death. Providers should familiarise themselves with the following guidance to help prevent this happening"

Appendix A advises use of audit tools for both doctors and nurses on tests for correct placement of a nasogastric tube.
See www.npsa.nhs.uk/nrls/alerts-and-directives/alerts/nasogastricfeeding-tubes

Event eight on the core list refers to 'Intravenous administration of mis-selected concentrated potassium chloride' .

It relates to:

"All care settings." (op cit)

Appendix A of the framework document states:

"Mis-selection of concentrated potassium chloride for intravenous administration for a flush or instead of the correct medication can have fatal effects. Providers should be aware of the following national advice to reduce the risk of this happening"

Appendix A refers to an NPSA alert that:

"recommends withdrawal of concentrated solutions from clinical areas other than defined critical care environments, and the use of prepared-in-pharmacy or bought solutions in standard diluted forms."

See www.npsa.nhs.uk/patientsafety/alerts-and-directives/alerts/potassium-chloride-concentrate

If events falling into the above categories should involve any death, the CI should ensure they take into account the 'never event' process that will be instigated. For more information on this see the document itself and also section 9.05.2.1 above.

Although the never events are perceived as likely to occur in a particular care setting they might occur in other care settings and if they do then CIs need to be aware that the never event reporting procedure should be followed.

10.03 Deaths in dental surgeries or following dental treatment

Deaths in dental surgeries or following dental treatment are comparatively rare (anecdotal). However a patient may have received medical intervention treatment at that surgery.

There may have been surgery or tooth extraction with subsequent unexpected haemorrhaging; anaesthetic with an unexpected reaction. A patient may have been sent home with a prescription from the dentist for antibiotics to which there has been a reaction such as anaphylactic shock.

Again, such deaths as these will usually be reported straight to the ME office as a death in the community. It will only when the family advises that there was a recent visit to the dentist, and the CMI investigates further, that any concern is likely to arise. Then the death will be referred on to the Coroner.

10.03.1 Specific investigation guidelines for an inquest – over and above the generic checklist

10.03.1.1 Circumstances

- Had there been any procedure or surgery?
  If so describe fully; had the dentist performed this procedure/surgery before? Were there any unexpected events during the procedure/surgery?
- What is the usual risk level involved in this sort of procedure/surgery? Was it raised for any reason? E.g. the pre-existing condition of the patient?
- Is it possible that there has been an adverse reaction to any anaesthetic? If so full details of the anaesthetic drugs, amounts and their effects will be needed
- Did the deceased have any previously diagnosed diseases injuries or illnesses that would have knowingly increased the risk of this procedure? E.g. was there a pre-existing cardiac condition? Was the patient on Warfarin or other anti-thrombolytic drugs?
- Were there additional complications found during the procedure/surgery that were previously unforeseen?
- Was the procedure / surgery elective or emergency?
- Were there any previously known allergies?
- Was the patient sent home with antibiotics to take later? Were any checks made to see if the patient had previously had that antibiotic (or one from the family of antibiotics)? How long previously? Were any checks made to see if there had been any adverse reaction? With whom were these checks made? E.g. the patient themselves or another family member

10.03.1.2 The time

- Did the person die in the surgery itself? Or outside? Or later e.g. at home?

10.03.1.3 Actions

- Seize any potential evidence – e.g. equipment / drugs
- Take photographs of equipment before moved (if possible)
- Seize any dental notes & photocopy them immediately
- Consider seizing equipment if necessary

10.03.1.4 Statements

It is unlikely that the CI will have a pre-existing working relationship with the dentist and their staff.

As each individual case varies so will the witnesses from whom statements will be needed. They may include (but may not be limited to) any of the following:

- Dentist
- Any dental nurse involved in the surgery / procedure
- Anyone else with any relevant knowledge – e.g. reception staff
- Family or other who knows what happened after the patient left the dentist surgery

10.03.2 'Never events' and dentists' surgeries

Dental surgeries are specifically not included in the core list of 'never events' (see section 9.05.2.1 above):

"Dentistry is to be excluded for the first phase." (op cit)

10.04 Deaths whilst under the care of the ambulance service

If a person dies in the community, the first medical attendance is quite often from the local ambulance service. In some instances the patient has already died and the ambulance service is unable to carry out any treatment and the staff verifies the fact of death.

In some instances the ambulance service are able to carry out treatment, the extent of which depends on the grade of the staff in attendance, with paramedics being more highly qualified than technicians and able to perform more procedures and give more drugs.

In some instances the ambulance will carry out this treatment at the place to which they were called. In other instances they will convey the decease to the local Accident and Emergency Department with treatment in progress en route.

10.04.1 Specific investigation guidelines for an inquest – over and above the generic checklist

10.04.1.1 Circumstances
- What were the circumstances?
- What was the initial call received by the ambulance service?
- Is it possible that there has been an adverse reaction to the anaesthetic? If so full details of the anaesthetic drugs, amounts and their effects will be needed
- Was the deceased previously known to the ambulance service? If so for what reason? Regular calls? Hoax calls? Inappropriate calls? Genuine calls?

10.04.1.2 The time
- Was someone with the patient when they died?
- If not – how long is it since they were last checked and alive?

10.04.1.3 Actions
- Seize any tape recordings of calls to and from the ambulance service and the crews
- Seize the ambulance crew record sheet and the statement of life extinct
- Obtain copies of any records relating to previous calls relating to this patient
- Obtain copy of the ambulance service policy about response to such an incident, covering both target times and actions to be taken

10.04.1.4 Statements

The existing working relationship that the CIs will have with the ambulance personnel they encounter at death scenes may help facilitate access to all necessary areas.

As each individual case varies so will the witnesses from whom statements will be needed. They may include (but may not be limited to) any of the following:

- All ambulance crew personnel
- Ambulance call centre staff (if relevant)
- Ambulance service managers (if relevant)

10.04.2 CQC and ambulance services

The CQC website stated in July 2009:

"We have the power to carry out investigations of NHS trusts if we have evidence that suggests a serious problem that may be putting patients at risk." www.cqc.org.uk

This includes ambulance service NHS Trusts (see section 9.05.1 above). There would need to be liaison between the CI and the CQC if there has been any investigation by them into a death involving an ambulance trust.

11

DEATHS IN SECONDARY HEALTHCARE SETTINGS

11.01 Introduction

This chapter concentrates on aspects specifically relevant to deaths in secondary healthcare settings and should be read in conjunction with Chapter 9 which is generic for all deaths in healthcare settings. See also Chapter 1 for more information on the proposed death certification process as contained in the Coroners and Justice Bill and in the DH programme overview paper 2008 on the process of death certification (op cit).

Deaths in secondary healthcare include deaths which arise from hospitals; residential care homes; nursing homes.

11.02 Deaths in Hospitals

These deaths will often be reported straight to the ME office and may be dealt with entirely within the ME system. They may be reported by the Bereavement Officer or via the staff in the Accident and Emergency Department where applicable, depending on local arrangements.

On many occasions the patient will have been seen by a doctor in hospital who is able to issue the MCCD and after scrutiny the ME will accept the causes of death without difficulty. There would be no referral to the Coroner and no post mortem examination.

However if there is any concern, either from the patient's family, or from the ME, the death will be referred on to the Coroner.

11.02.1 Family concerns

The family may be dissatisfied with the treatment that the deceased had been receiving from the doctor and make their concerns known. The MEO will make initial enquiries into the concerns. The ME will discuss the matter with the family and the cause of their concerns may be allayed and an MCCD issued. However, they concerns may not be allayed and the ME's office will refer the death to the Coroner for a post mortem examination.

The results of such an examination may then allay the family's concerns. They may show that the doctor's professional judgment and treatment of the patient was accurate. They may show that there was an underlying illness or disease of which the doctor was unaware. However, the matter may need to progress to an inquest investigation and hearing.

11.02.2 Doctors' concerns

On occasions a hospital doctor cannot state the cause of death with any degree of certainty. Perhaps there were many existing co-pathologies and the doctor cannot be sure which the primary cause was. Perhaps the patient had died before investigations could establish what illness or disease the patient was suffering from and the cause of death is therefore not known. Following such deaths there will have been discussion between the doctor and the ME's office but there may need to be a referral to the Coroner for a post mortem examination to establish the cause of death.

11.02.3 Recent operation or procedure

There may have been a recent operation or invasive procedure. Indeed the patient may have died in the anaesthetic room pre-operatively (for example as an adverse reaction to an anaesthetic); "on the table" in an operating theatre (for example if an aneurysm ruptures); in the recovery room post-operatively; in the radiology department where radiological procedures take place (for example during a barium enema).

Most Coroners require any such case to proceed to post mortem examination, to establish that the death was despite the operation or procedure, and not caused by it.

11.02.4 Had not seen the doctor

The patient may not yet have been seen by a doctor. For example a patient may have been triaged by a nurse in the Accident and Emergency Department but not yet seen the doctor. It is quite likely that many such cases will require referral to the Coroner from the ME's office. A similar circumstance might arise in the Out-Patients Department.

11.02.5 Specific investigation guidelines for an inquest – over and above the generic checklist

11.02.5.1 Circumstances

- What had the patient been doing in the hospital?
- Which part of the hospital were they in? For example: Accident and Emergency; mainstream ward (medical or surgical); theatres; radiology department; initial assessment unit; out-patient department; day surgery department
- Had there been any procedure or surgery?
  If so describe fully; had the doctor performed this procedure/surgery before? Were there any unexpected events during the procedure/surgery?
- What is the usual risk level involved in this sort of procedure/surgery? Was it raised for any reason? E.g. the pre-existing condition of the patient?
- Is it possible that an error was made during a procedure?
- Is it possible that there has been an adverse reaction to any anaesthetic? If so full details of the anaesthetic drugs, amounts and their effects will be needed
- Did the deceased have any previously diagnosed diseases injuries or illnesses that would have knowingly increased the risk of this procedure? E.g. was there a pre-existing cardiac condition? Was the patient on Warfarin or other anti-thrombolytic drugs?
- Were there additional complications found during the procedure/surgery that were previously unforeseen?
- Was the procedure/surgery elective or emergency?
- Were there any previously known allergies?
- Had there been a fall within the hospital premises/grounds?

11.02.5.2 Actions

- Seize any potential evidence – e.g. equipment/drugs
- Take photographs of equipment before moved (if possible)
- Seize any medical notes & photocopy them immediately
- Obtain a copy of any accident or incident book entry and any RIDDOR form submitted by the Trust
- Obtain copies of all relevant care plans and risk assessments
- Obtain a copy of any relevant NICE guidelines
- Obtain a copy of the Trust's internal investigative report

11.02.5.3 Statements

As each individual case varies so will the witnesses from whom statements will be needed. They may include (but may not be limited to) any of the following:

- Doctor who performed procedure/surgery
- Any other staff member who was present
- Any other health practitioner who was with the patient
- Any other patients or family members who witnessed events

11.02.6 'Never events' and hospitals

Events one, two, three, four, seven and eight on the core list of 'never events' would apply if the 'event' had occurred at a hospital (see section 9.05.2.1 above):

Event one on the core list refers to 'wrong site surgery' which is described as:

"A surgical intervention performed on the wrong site (for example wrong knee, wrong eye, wrong patient, wrong limb, or wrong organ); the incident is detected after the operation and the patient requires further surgery, on the correct site, and/or may have complications following the wrong surgery." (op cit)

It specifically relates to:

"Organisations that provide major, minor and/or day case surgery."

Appendix A of the framework document states:

"Operating on the wrong site can have devastating consequences for patients."
(op cit)

Appendix A advises implementation of guidance from the World Health Organisation and the use of a surgical safety checklist to prevent wrong site surgery.
See www.npsa.nhs.uk/nrls/alerts-and-directives/alerts/safer-surgery-alert

It also advises use of standard wristbands to reduce the possibility of the wrong patient receiving the surgery.
See www.npsa.nhs.uk/nrls/alerts-and-directives/notices/wristbands

Event two on the core list refers to 'retained instrument post-operation' which is described as:

"One or more instruments are unintentionally retained following an operative procedure, and an operation or other invasive procedure is needed to remove this, and/or there are complications to the patient arising from its continued presence. This Never Event does not include interventional radiology or cardiology procedures, and the definition of instrument does not include guide wires, screws, swabs or other similar material." (op cit)

It specifically relates to:

"Organisations that provide major, minor and/or day case surgery."

Appendix A of the framework document states:

"Unintentionally retained instruments are a potential cause of complications and repeat surgery. Most providers will have developed their own local policies based on available advice."

Appendix A refers to various advice documents which CIs can access if the need arises.

Event three on the core list refers to 'wrong route administration of chemotherapy' which is described as:

"Intravenous or other chemotherapy (for example, vincristine) that is correctly prescribed but administered via the wrong route (usually into the intrathecal space)" (op cit)

It relates to:

"Acute care settings."

Appendix A of the framework document states:

"Cancer drugs such as vincristine continue to be given occasionally via the wrong route worldwide, sometimes resulting in paralysis or death of a patient."

Appendix A refers to various advice documents which CIs can access if the need arises.

Event four on the core list refers to 'misplaced naso or orogastric tube not detected prior to use' which is described as:

"Naso or orogastric tube placed in the respiratory tract rather than the gastrointestinal tract and not detected prior to commencing feeding or other use.." *(op cit)*

It relates to:

"All care settings."

Appendix A of the framework document states:

"There is a risk that nasogastric or orogastric feeding tubes may be inserted in a lung or bronchus instead of the stomach, resulting in potentially serious harm and/or death. Providers should familiarise themselves with the following guidance to help prevent this happening"

Appendix A advises use of audit tools for both doctors and nurses on tests for correct placement of a nasogastric tube.
See www.npsa.nhs.uk/nrls/alerts-and-directives/alerts/nasogastricfeeding-tubes

Event seven on the core list refers to 'In-hospital maternal death from post-partum haemorrhage after elective caesarean section' which is described as:

"In-hospital death of a mother as a result of a haemorrhage following elective caesarean section, excluding cases where imaging has identified placenta accrete" *(op cit)*

It specifically relates to:

"Acute care maternity services"

Appendix A of the framework document states:

"obstetric haemorrhage remains a problem in terms of both morbidity and mortality. Providers should be aware of applicable guidelines before and after caesarean section to prevent women from dying from haemorrhage, particularly after an elective procedure."

Appendix A refers to various advice documents which CIs can access if the need arises including the WHO Surgical Safety Checklist (as above).

Event eight on the core list refers to 'Intravenous administration of mis-selected concentrated potassium chloride'.

It relates to:

"All care settings." (op cit)

Appendix A of the framework document states:

"Mis-selection of concentrated potassium chloride for intravenous administration for a flush or instead of the correct medication can have fatal effects. Providers should be aware of the following national advice to reduce the risk of this happening"

Appendix A refers to an NPSA alert that:

"recommends withdrawal of concentrated solutions from clinical areas other than defined critical care environments, and the use of prepared-in-pharmacy or bought solutions in standard diluted forms."

See www.npsa.nhs.uk/patientsafety/alerts-and-directives/alerts/potassium-chloride-concentrate

If events falling into the above categories should involve any death, the CI should ensure they take into account the 'never event' process that will be instigated. For more information on this see the document itself and also section 9.05.2.1 above.

Although the never events are perceived as likely to occur in a particular care setting they might occur in other care settings and if they do then CIs need to be aware that the never event reporting procedure should be followed.

See also the DH leaflet: When a Patient Dies: Advice on Developing Bereavement Services in the NHS (2005) for guidance on the procedures that should be in place in hospitals for when someone dies.

11.02.7 CQC

The CQC website stated in July 2009:

"We have the power to carry out investigations of NHS trusts if we have evidence that suggests a serious problem that may be putting patients at risk."
www.cqc.org.uk

There would need to be liaison between the CI and the CQC if they have conducted any investigation into a death in a hospital.

11.03 Deaths in residential care homes

These deaths will often be reported straight to the ME's office and may be dealt with entirely within the ME system. They will usually be reported by the patient's GP. On many occasions the patient will have been seen by the GP who is able to issue the MCCD and after scrutiny the ME will accept the causes of death without difficulty. There would be no referral to the Coroner and no post mortem examination.

However if there is any concern, either from the patient's family, or from the ME, the death will be referred on to the Coroner.

11.03.1 Family concerns

The family may be dissatisfied with the treatment that the deceased had been receiving and make their concerns known. The MEO will make initial enquiries into the concerns. The ME will discuss the matter with the family and the cause of their concerns may be allayed and an MCCD issued. However, they concerns may not be allayed and the ME's Office will refer the death to the Coroner for a post mortem examination.

The results of such an examination may then allay the family's concerns. They may show that the doctor's professional judgment and treatment of the patient was accurate. They may show that there was an underlying illness or disease of which the doctor was unaware. However, the matter may need to progress to an inquest investigation and hearing.

11.03.2 Doctors' concerns

On occasions a GP cannot state the cause of death with any degree of certainty. Perhaps there were many existing co-pathologies and the doctor cannot be sure which the primary cause was. Perhaps the patient was being investigated but died before investigations could establish what illness or disease the patient was suffering from and the cause of death is therefore not known. Following such deaths there will have been discussion between the doctor and the ME's office but there may need to be a referral to the Coroner for a post mortem examination to establish the cause of death.

11.03.3 Recent operation or procedure

There may have been a recent operation or invasive procedure (for example in a hospital as an out-patient or prior to discharge to the residential care home). Most Coroners require any such case to proceed to post mortem examination, to establish that the death was despite the operation or procedure, and not caused by it.

11.03.4 Had not seen the doctor

The patient may not have been seen by a doctor within the required time period. This has traditional been taken as fourteen days because of current legislative requirements under cremation legislation (hence the "14 day rule").

11.03.5 Recent fall or incident

Many residents in residential care homes are elderly or frail, hence being in the care home at all. Being elderly or frail makes one more prone to falls for many reasons, such as underlying illness or disease, poor eyesight, reduced mobility. If there has been a fall immediately prior to a death or in the fairly recent past, the death is likely to be referred to the Coroner for a post mortem examination to be sure that the death occurred despite the fall rather than because of it. Of course if a fall or other incident has lead to the death there will need to be a coroner's inquest investigation and hearing.

11.03.6 Specific investigation guidelines for an inquest – over and above the generic checklist

11.03.6.1 Circumstances

- How long had the resident been at that home? Had they moved there recently? Were they unfamiliar with their surroundings?
- What was the physical and medical condition of the deceased?
- What medication was prescribed? Was it being taken appropriately?
- Had there been a fall or other incident?

11.03.6.2 Actions

- Seize any potential evidence – e.g. equipment / drugs
- Take photographs of any relevant areas in the home
- Seize any notes & photocopy them immediately
- Obtain copies of all relevant care plans and risk assessments
- Obtain a copy of any accident or incident book entry and any RIDDOR form completed
- Obtain a copy of any medication sheet
- If appropriate seize medications*
- Establish staffing levels at the time of any incident surrounding a death**
- Obtain a copy of the relevant procedures within the home
- Obtain a copy of any relevant NICE guidelines
- Obtain a copy of the last two CSCI reports into the home

*In the 2003 DH document "Care Homes for Older People: National Minimum Standards" it states:

"When a service user dies, medicines should be retained for a period of seven days in case there is a coroner's inquest." (op cit para 9.11)

** *In the 2003 DH document "Care Homes for Older People: National Minimum Standards" Standard 27 states:*

"27.2 A recorded staff rota showing which staff are on duty at any time during the day and night and in what capacity is kept.

27.3 The ratios of care staff to service users must be determined according to the assessed needs of residents, and a system operated for calculating staff numbers required, in accordance with guidance recommended by the Department of Health.

27.4 Additional staff are on duty at peak times of activity during the day.

27.5 There are waking night staff on duty in numbers that reflect the numbers and needs of service users and the layout of the home. In care homes providing nursing this includes registered nurse(s)." (op cit)

The Care Home Regulations 2001 require certain records to be kept in a care home in respect of each 'service user' including:

"(i) a record of all medicines kept in the care home for the service user, and the date on which they were administered to the service user;

(j) a record of any accident affecting the service user in the care home and of any other

incident in the care home which is detrimental to the health or welfare of the service user, which record shall include the nature, date and time of the accident or incident, whether medical treatment was required and the name of the persons who were respectively in charge of the care home and supervising the service user;

......

(n) a record of incidence of pressure sores and of treatment provided to the service user;

(o) a record of falls and of treatment provided to the service user;

(p) a record of any physical restraint used on the service user;

A copy of correspondence relating to each service user."

The Care Home Regulations 2001 also require other records to be kept in a care home including:

A copy of the duty roster of persons working at the care home, and a record of whether the roster was actually worked.

12. A record of any of the following events that occur in the care home -
(a) any accident;
(b) any incident which is detrimental to the health or welfare of a service user
13. Records of the food provided for service users in sufficient detail to enable any person inspecting the record to determine whether the diet is satisfactory, in relation to nutrition and otherwise, and of any special diets prepared for individual service users.

It follows that all of these documents will be available to the Coroner through his CI if necessary following the death of any 'service user' and the CI should be aware of this and ask for any relevant documents.

11.03.6.3 Statements

As each individual case varies so will the witnesses from whom statements will be needed. They may include (but may not be limited to) any of the following:

- Owner or manager of the home to cover pre-admission assessment of the resident, noting any relevant medical or physical conditions
- Owner or manager of the home to cover required staffing levels; actual staffing levels
- Person who last saw the resident alive including where and when and how he/she was at that time
- Person who found the resident collapsed or dead including where and when
- Any other health practitioner who was with the patient
- Any other patients or family members who witnessed events

See also Appendices 10, 11, 12 and 13 for specific checklists concerning falls; head injuries; Warfarin; pressure ulcers.

See also the DH document: When a Patient Dies: Advice on Developing Bereavement Services in the NHS (2005). Section 15 and 16 state:

"Independent providers of care face the same issues in the provision of bereavement services as does the NHS. For example, the National Minimum

Standards (NMS) for care homes for older people set out the regulations on all aspects of care that must be met for individual care homes to legally operate. The NMS contain standards on death and dying with the stated outcome as:
Service users are assured that at the time of their death, staff will treat them and their family with care, sensitivity and respect." (op cit)

Standard 11 states that the following should be met:
11.2 That policies and procedures for handling dying and death are in place and observed by staff.
11.8 That palliative care, practical assistance and advice and bereavement counselling are provided by trained professionals/specialist agencies if the service user wishes." (op cit)

11.03.7 'Never events' and residential care homes

Event four on the core list refers to 'misplaced naso or orogastric tube not detected prior to use' which is described as:

"Naso or orogastric tube placed in the respiratory tract rather than the gastrointestinal tract and not detected prior to commencing feeding or other use.." (op cit)

It relates to:

"All care settings."

Appendix A of the framework document states:

"There is a risk that nasogastric or orogastric feeding tubes may be inserted in a lung or bronchus instead of the stomach, resulting in potentially serious harm and/or death. Providers should familiarise themselves with the following guidance to help prevent this happening"

Appendix A advises use of audit tools for both doctors and nurses on tests for correct placement of a nasogastric tube.

See www.npsa.nhs.uk/nrls/alerts-and-directives/alerts/nasogastricfeeding-tubes

Although the never events are perceived as likely to occur in a particular care setting they might occur in other care settings and if they do then CIs need to be aware that the never event reporting procedure should be followed.

11.04 Deaths in nursing homes

These deaths will often be reported straight to the ME's office and may be dealt with entirely within the ME system. They may be reported by the GP or on occasions via the funeral directors. This latter may arise if a death occurred out of hours and the staff expected that the GP would issue an MCCD and so arranged the funeral directors' attendance without any death certificate. A nurse from the nursing home, or a doctor from the out of hours doctors' cooperative will have verified the fact of death.

All of the text above relating to deaths in residential care homes relate to nursing homes. However nursing homes are required to provide qualified nursing staff and there is an expectation that they will provide nursing care. Most residents of nursing homes are in that particular home because they have nursing requirements. However it should be noted that this is not always the case and some privately funded residents may live in a nursing home even if they do not have nursing needs. For example a husband and wife move into a nursing home together as one of them needs nursing care. That person subsequently dies and the remaining resident wishes to stay in their "home". No matter whether the resident requires nursing care, there is still a minimum level of nursing staff and a minimum ration of qualified : unqualified staff in any nursing home.

11.04.1 Specific investigation guidelines for an inquest – over and above the generic checklist and the text relating to residential care homes

11.04.1.1 Actions

- Obtain a copy of any action plans and reviews thereof
- Obtain copies of all relevant care plans and risk assessments

The Care Home Regulations 2001 require certain records to be kept in a care home in respect of each 'service user'. These are mentioned at section 11.03.6.2 and apply equally to a nursing home. IN addition the home is required to keep:

"(k) a record of any nursing provided to the service user, including a record of his condition and any treatment or surgical intervention; details of any specialist communications needs of the service user and methods of communication that may be appropriate to the service user;
(m) details of any plan relating to the service user in respect of medication, nursing, specialist health care or nutrition. "
It follows that all of these documents will be available to the Coroner through his CI if necessary following the death of any 'service user' and the CI should be aware of this and ask for any relevant documents.

11.04.1.2 Statements
As each individual case varies so will the witnesses from whom statements will be needed. They may include (but may not be limited to) any of the following:

- Owner or manager or matron of the home to cover pre-admission assessment of the resident, noting any relevant medical or physical conditions
- Owner or manager or matron of the home to cover required staffing levels; actual staffing levels at relevant times; ratio of qualified to unqualified staff required at relevant times

11.04.2 'Never events' and nursing homes
Event four on the core list refers to 'misplaced naso or orogastric tube not detected prior to use' which is described as:

"Naso or orogastric tube placed in the respiratory tract rather than the gastrointestinal tract and not detected prior to commencing feeding or other use.."
(op cit)

It relates to:

"All care settings."

Appendix A of the framework document states:

"There is a risk that nasogastric or orogastric feeding tubes may be inserted in a lung or bronchus instead of the stomach, resulting in potentially serious harm and/or death. Providers should familiarise themselves with the following guidance to help prevent this happening"

Appendix A advises use of audit tools for both doctors and nurses on tests for correct placement of a nasogastric tube. See www.npsa.nhs.uk/nrls/alerts-and-directives/alerts/nasogastricfeeding-tubes

Although the never events are perceived as likely to occur in a particular care setting they might occur in other care settings and if they do then CIs need to be aware that the never event reporting procedure should be followed.

11.05 Miscellaneous

See also Appendices 10, 11, 12 and 13 for specific checklists concerning falls; head injuries; Warfarin; pressure ulcers.

See also the DH leaflet: When a Patient Dies: Advice on Developing Bereavement Services in the NHS (2005). Section 15 and 16 state:

"Independent providers of care face the same issues in the provision of bereavement services as does the NHS. For example, the National Minimum Standards (NMS) for care homes for older people set out the regulations on all aspects of care that must be met for individual care homes to legally operate. The NMS contain standards on death and dying with the stated outcome as:
Service users are assured that at the time of their death, staff will treat them and their family with care, sensitivity and respect.

Standard 11 states that the following should be met:

11.3 That policies and procedures for handling dying and death are in place and observed by staff.

11.9 That palliative care, practical assistance and advice and bereavement counselling are provided by trained professionals/specialist agencies if the service user wishes." (op cit)

12

DEATHS IN PALLIATIVE HEALTHCARE SETTINGS

12.01 Introduction

This chapter concentrates on aspects specifically relevant to deaths in palliative healthcare settings and should be read in conjunction with Chapter 9 which is generic for all deaths in healthcare settings. See also Chapter 1 for more information on the proposed death certification process as contained in the Coroners and Justice Bill and in the DH programme overview paper 2008 on the process of death certification (op cit).

12.02 Deaths in Hospices

Under the proposed system most of these deaths will be reported to the ME office and dealt with entirely within the ME system.

This is because the hospice doctor will usually have been in attendance within the last few days and will have a clear idea of the cause of death for the MCCD.

12.02.1 Family concerns

It is rare that the family will have concerns when a relative has been treated within the hospice situation (anecdotal). However if they do then actions and records as discussed in the previous two chapters may apply if relevant. For example seizing of records or equipment and taking of statements.

Any family concerns are likely to be aligned to fear of "mercy killing" by a healthcare professional and the police would need to be involved early on (see also Chapter 1).

12.02.2 Industrial disease

The most usual reasons for referral surround industrial disease and those mainly arise from asbestos related deaths such as mesothelioma. In some parts of the country other industrial diseases may appear more frequently, such as silicosis; farmers lung; tuberculosis (for example in a mortuary worker or pathologist). See The Social Security (Industrial Injuries) (Prescribed Diseases) Regulations 1985 for a full list of those diseases which, if leading to death, would require referral to the Coroner.

The reason for referral is that such deaths will require a box to be ticked on the front of the MCCD, indicating that:

"The death might have been due to or contributed to by the employment followed at some time by the deceased."

The action taken by the Coroner following such a referral varies around England and Wales. Some Coroners do not consider it necessary to hold an inquest when a death is attributed to asbestos. Others insist on a post mortem examination and if the word "asbestos" appears anywhere in part 1a, 1b or 1c of the MCCD an investigative inquest will need to be held.

The requirement to refer a death to a Coroner also applies for any potentially industrial disease related death even if not in the hospice situation.

12.02.3 Specific investigation guidelines for an inquest – over and above the generic checklist

12.02.3.1 Circumstances

- What were the underlying diseases / pathologies
- Is there any suspected or known past occupational link? If so what?

12.02.3.2 Actions

- Obtain medical notes for any relevant correspondence; test and investigation results

- Obtain all documentation relating to any claim on the government or a former employer or their insurer for compensation

12.02.3.3 Statements

As each individual case varies so will the witnesses from whom statements will be needed. They may include (but may not be limited to) any of the following:

- Family as to occupation al exposure and work history with dates, job titles and what the roles involved
- Solicitor as to details of any claims made (whether or not still in progress and whether or not successful)

See also Appendix 14 for a specific checklist concerning asbestos related deaths for use in those areas where the Coroner will require an investigation.

12.02.4 Trauma

The other most likely reason for referral from a hospice arises when there has at some past stage been a traumatic incident, for example a road traffic collision which has resulted in a severe head injury or persistent vegetative state. Such scenarios will often involve hospice care and hospice doctors know that there is a possibility that the Coroner will need to hold an investigative inquest into the original incident that has contributed to the person's death.

12.02.4.1 Specific investigation guidelines for an inquest – over and above the generic checklist

12.02.4.1.1 Circumstances

- What was the original incident?

12.02.4.1.2 Actions

- Obtain full details of original incident
- Obtain medical notes for any relevant correspondence; test and investigation results
- Obtain all documentation relating to any claim for insurance

- Establish whether anyone was dealt with through the criminal courts (e.g. for driving offences)

12.02.4.1.3 Statements

As each individual case varies so will the witnesses from whom statements will be needed. They may include (but may not be limited to) any of the following:

- Family as to details of original incident
- Any police-obtained statements if there was a criminal prosecution
- Solicitor as to details of any civil claim

See also Appendix 10 for a specific checklist concerning falls and Appendix 11 for a specific checklist concerning head injuries and chapter five for road traffic collisions.

12.02.5 'Never events' and hospices

Event three on the core list refers to 'wrong route administration of chemotherapy' which is described as:

"Intravenous or other chemotherapy (for example, vincristine) that is correctly prescribed but administered via the wrong route (usually into the intrathecal space)" (op cit)

It relates to:

"Acute care settings."

Appendix A of the framework document states:

"Cancer drugs such as vincristine continue to be given occasionally via the wrong route worldwide, sometimes resulting in paralysis or death of a patient."

Appendix A refers to various advice documents which CIs can access if the need arises.

Event four on the core list refers to 'misplaced naso or orogastric tube not detected prior to use' which is described as:

"Naso or orogastric tube placed in the respiratory tract rather than the gastrointestinal tract and not detected prior to commencing feeding or other use.."
(op cit)

It relates to:

"All care settings."

Appendix A of the framework document states:

"There is a risk that nasogastric or orogastric feeding tubes may be inserted in a lung or bronchus instead of the stomach, resulting in potentially serious harm and/or death. Providers should familiarise themselves with the following guidance to help prevent this happening"

Appendix A advises use of audit tools for both doctors and nurses on tests for correct placement of a nasogastric tube.
See www.npsa.nhs.uk/nrls/alerts-and-directives/alerts/nasogastricfeeding-tubes

Event eight on the core list refers to 'Intravenous administration of mis-selected concentrated potassium chloride'.

It relates to:

"All care settings." *(op cit)*

Appendix A of the framework document states:

"Mis-selection of concentrated potassium chloride for intravenous administration for a flush or instead of the correct medication can have fatal effects. Providers should be aware of the following national advice to reduce the risk of this happening"

Appendix A refers to an NPSA alert that:

"recommends withdrawal of concentrated solutions from clinical areas other than defined critical care environments, and the use of prepared-in-pharmacy or bought solutions in standard diluted forms."

See www.npsa.nhs.uk/patientsafety/alerts-and-directives/alerts/potassium-chloride-concentrate

If events falling into the above categories should involve any death, the CI should ensure they take into account the 'never event' process that will be instigated. For more information on this see the document itself and also section 9.05.2.1 above.

Although the never events are perceived as likely to occur in a particular care setting they might occur in other care settings and if they do then CIs need to be aware that the never event reporting procedure should be followed.

12.02.6 CQC and hospices

The CQC website stated in July 2009:

"To help protect the public, many of the healthcare services offered by the independent sector must by law be registered with us." www.cqc.org.uk

This includes hospices. The website continues:

"Before we will register a healthcare provider, we check to make sure that they meet the Government's national minimum standards for independent healthcare. This includes looking at the quality of their treatment and services, and at the safety and cleanliness of their premises and equipment. We also check the staff's qualifications and skills, arrangements for further training and professional development, and the provider's procedures for handling any complaints. To make sure that registered providers maintain good standards of care, we check on their services each year." (op cit)

13

THE CORONER'S INVESTIGATOR & STATEMENT TAKING

13.01 Introduction

Statements are ways of recording the information that will help the Coroner reach an appropriate verdict at an inquest. They are also the method of recording the information outlined in preceding chapters for specific type of deaths. The CI should remember that witness statements may at some point be seen by the family or others close to the deceased. They may be read out in court. It exhibits sensitivity to refer to the deceased by name, as opposed to "the deceased". Similarly "he" rather than "the male" etc.

13.02 Recipients of statements

Initially and primarily a CI will be taking a statement for the Coroner and their investigation. However rules of disclosure being unclear, it is quite possible that a Coroner may disclose any statement to other individuals or organisations. Therefore statement makers should not be misled into thinking that the statement is only ever for the Coroner. If a statement is made subject to section 9 of the Criminal Justice Act 1967 (CJA) (see section 12.6 below) then it is possible for someone to incriminate themselves or open the door to perjury offences and this should not be ignored.

13.02.1 The Coroner

A CI should ideally know the sort of information the Coroner will want in the statement. Practically, this information can only be built up through working with that Coroner. Each Coroner is different and has different wants and dislikes. A rule of thumb for the CI is to think - if the Coroner were taking the statement - what would he want it to include?

13.02.2 The police

If evidence of a crime becomes apparent in a statement then the question of whether and how that information should be passed to the police will need to be resolved (under the Coroner's direction). If an investigation "changes status" (see section 1.15 above), then statements obtained will need to be copied to police.

13.02.3 Other agencies

Statements may be copied to other agencies under certain circumstances. For example in a death involving actual or potential electrocution, it may be that the electricity board will want to see the statement to consider whether prosecutions are appropriate. Similarly cases involving Health and Safety may involve statement transfer. CIs therefore have to bear this in mind when taking statements.

13.03 Who should take the statement?

13.03.1 The best

The best possible person to take the statement has to be the individual CI dealing with the case. The ability to pick up on cues and clues from witnesses needs an in-depth knowledge of the whole case. Such knowledge cannot all be passed effectively on to a third party. Thus the possibility of an intermediary missing and following up on a vital cue (and clue) exists. The government's position paper (2004) commented on statement taking:

"We see the coroner's officer as having a more clearly defined and consistent **investigative role** *(sic) than is often the case at present: going out to take statements from the next of kin or to visit scenes of death, where relevant. In this way, they could take over from the police many responsibilities in relation to non-suspicious deaths. Coroners' officers would need to continue to maintain close links with bereaved families throughout the death investigation process." (op cit paragraph 60)*

However there is one common exception to this scenario – with the child or vulnerable witness. There are specially trained police officers with skills and equipment able to take information from such people ensuring that the notion of truth is clearly understood, and without causing undue harm or anxiety to the witness. It is recommended that these experienced police officers are involved in the taking of such statements or information.

13.03.2 Other CIs

If an intermediary is necessary then a CI in the relevant area (if in England, Wales or Northern Ireland) can be asked to obtain the statement. They may have an appreciation of Coroners' statements, hearsay issues and of the possibility of individualities of Coroners. It is also possibly easier to first telephone a Coroner's Office and speak to a specific Investigator direct and discuss the case with him / her before sending the information request through. This may increase the chances of a "successful outcome".

13.03.3 Other officials

Asking a police officer in the relevant force area of the witness is a strategy that can be used. Such a statement request may need to be very specific to ensure the information that the particular Coroner requires is included.

However, there are some disadvantages with asking any other to take the statement as outlined below.

13.03.3.1 Omissions

Such persons are likely to omit information relevant to the inquest, simply through lack of regular contact with the Coroner – rather than because of any inadequacy or inability.

13.03.3.2 Logistic difficulty

Practically, asking another to take a statement is not an easy solution, relying as it does on another's good will and on a gap in their workload. Most police officers work shifts and are already pressured. As such they do not have time to deal with their own workload let alone carry out tasks on behalf of another. The situation is similar for other CIs.

13.04 Who to take statements from?

See section 2.11 for generic information on statements. See also chapters 3 - 12 on specific types of deaths in relation to additional statements and what extra information needs to be obtained.

There may be occasions when the CI's judgment is that a statement is not needed from a particular individual. This might be after discussion with that individual and establishing that there is no additional information to be added by this individual. However simply to tell a person offering to assist that their information is not needed might be seen as insensitive. Nevertheless, a line has to be drawn somewhere - without limitless resources. A resolution might be to explain that it is not clear that they have any additional evidence to provide, but if they would like to write their information down and send it in - of course they can.

13.05 What to include in a statement

13.05.1 Negative and positive

A Coroner is concerned with establishing the facts as far as possible and thus negative evidence is as valuable as positive.

Does the person think that it could be a suicide – if yes record why. If no, record why not. The current burden of proof for a suicide statement is such that if there are reasons why it should not be considered as a suicide, these need to be brought to the Coroner's attention. It is not the role of the CI to filter out information that does not fit their own opinion as to what has occurred.

Another example of positive and negative would be - did the person hear a noise or see something – or not?

Positive evidence might be to negate or support any potential explanation of events.

13.05.2 Hearsay

A Coroner is not bound by rules of hearsay in the same way that a criminal court is. Hearsay is advantageous to Coroners for many reasons. One is to overcome a scenario where one witness is unwilling or unable to supply information (see section 12.7 below). If there is a witness who can say that "Mark told me that Joanne had said to him that she wanted to go to sleep and never wake up", this should be recorded in this witness's statement. It may be that a statement is never obtained from Mark for some reason - but the information vital to the Coroner is not now lost.

Another important advantage of the hearsay leniency, is where the witness himself dies, after having given the statement and before appearing in court. This need not be a problem for the Coroner as rule 37(5) of the Coroners Rules 1984 states:

"A coroner may admit as evidence at an inquest any document made by a deceased person if he is of the opinion that the contents of the document are relevant to the purposes of the inquest."

The dilemma for the CI then is to try and anticipate every possible eventuality in relation to a statement being taken and to balance the information that is included therein.

13.05.3 Duplication

It follows from hearsay that it is better to have the same piece of information recorded from a number of witnesses, confirming the overall picture, than for it to be missed altogether.

13.05.4 Inconsistency

As with statements from a number of witnesses in any environment, inconsistencies are to be expected. A CI should not be alarmed by this, and should record what they are told. It would be very strange indeed if all witnesses to a road traffic collision were to see and recall exactly the same. Coroners, as with Magistrates or Judges in other environments, might suspect collusion.

A CI should be aware of inconsistencies and probe to see if they are resolvable. Inconsistency is another reason for the same CI taking all the statements in any given investigation.

Different inconsistencies may cause different levels of probing. Consider an example of two people seen to jump off a cliff. The fact that one person saw them jump together, holding hands, while another says there was a clear gap of at least four seconds between the two jumping while a third saw one push the other off and then jump themselves - such discrepancies would require probing and resolution. The fact that one witness thought a man found hanging was wearing a blue shirt, while another recalled the shirt being green - should be recorded but is not necessarily of significance (although under some circumstances it may be).

Apart from the case where inconsistency raises suspicion and the police need to be alerted it will be for the Coroner to determine the relevance of any inconsistencies.

13.05.5 Exhibit production

The statement is the clearest way of introducing exhibits into an inquest. The general rule is that the first person to mention an item produces it as their exhibit. Thus the finder of a "suicide note" would exhibit in their statement, including details of where they found it. If the "note" is subsequently shown to another to identify the hand-writing, that other would not exhibit the note as their exhibit – avoiding duplication of references in a number of statements.

However on many occasions CIs will produce exhibits with their own reference number. For example, the finder of a rucksack at the top of cliffs raises the alarm and leaves the scene – without leaving their details. They cannot produce the exhibit – but it needs to be produced.

CIs who attend the scene of a death and seize the medication (as discussed in sections 1.08.5.4, 1.09.5 and 2.10 above) will produce the items listed as their exhibit. CIs who attend a scene of a death and take photographs will produce the album of photographs as their exhibit.

13.06 Section 9 CJA statements (Criminal Justice Act 1967)

At present there is no requirement for the Coroner to have information passed to him in the form of a statement. Information can reach the Coroner in handwritten letter form. Indeed such information does not even need to be signed by the maker. There is no requirement for the Coroner that any statement should have a section 9 CJA rider attached to it.

There are however good reasons why a statement should be taken subject to section 9, and for it to be signed:

- A Coroner still has a power to deal with matters of contempt and a false statement could fall within that ambit
- Perjury is an offence that can be committed in any court, including the Coroner's. A section 9 statement could support a charge of perjury. However the CI will need to give the appropriate warning for the section 9 to be valid
- A Coroner may consider the offence of attempting to pervert the course of justice (where an inquest is "justice")
- Making a false statement may also amount to the common law offence of obstructing a Coroner
- A signature is evidence of the maker's identity

13.06.1 Statement maker not in court

A reason for the statement to be as full as possible and signed by the maker is that there are any number of reasons why that person may not make it to a formal hearing (see for example section 13.5.2 above). Should the nature of inquests change and there be less personal appearance by statement makers then the status of the statement may well be increased. The Coroner does not call every statement maker to the inquest as a witness. Rule 37 Coroners Rules 1984 concerns the Coroner's power to produce documentary evidence.

13.06.2 Police headed statement form or other

There is a separate debate as to whether any statement for a Coroner's investigation needs to be obtained on a police statement form (if the CI is employed by a police authority) or on a Coroner's form devised for the purpose. In some jurisdictions where CIs are employed by the police the statement forms used are those of the local police force, with the police crest and name on the top. In others, Coroners have created their own forms – replacing the crest and name with their coronial details. This latter approach may have the effect of appearing more independent from the police which is beneficial. Similarly it may reduce potential problems of ownership of the statement. In those areas where police forms are used, CIs can find themselves in the awkward situation of police applying pressure for a statement which the Coroner has ruled should not be released to them. What is the CI to do in these circumstances? Preferable not to be in that situation at all.

Where CIs are no longer employed by police then that debate should cease. What format the statement layout were to take would be a matter for any new employer.

13.07 Powers to require a statement

There is no power yet available to a CI to require anyone to provide a statement for a Coroner's investigation.

However, the Coroners and Justice Bill enables a coroner to require a person to give evidence or provide documents for the purposes of an investigation. Schedule 4 Paragraph 1 (2):

"A senior coroner who is conducting an investigation under this Part may by notice require a person within such period as the coroner thinks reasonable:-
a) to provide evidence to the senior coroner, about any matters specified in the notice, in the form of a written statement
b) to produce any documents in the custody or under the control of the person which relate to a matter that is relevant to the investigation." (op cit)

However there are limitations:

"A person may not be required to give, produce or provide any evidence or document under Paragraph 1 if-

(a) he or she could not be required to do so in civil proceedings in a court in England and Wales, or
(b) the requirement would be incompatible with a Community obligation."
(Schedule 4 Paragraph 2 (1) (op cit))

Most witnesses will provide the information the Coroner requires without any problems. The vast majority of the population want to be helpful in any situation.

However, there is a segment of population that will not want to be helpful. The Coroner can deal with this by issuing a witness summons and calling the witness to the inquest. No statement needs to have been taken in advance.

"A senior coroner may by notice in writing require any person in England and Wales to attend at a time and place stated in the notice:-
a) to give evidence at an inquest" *(Draft Coroner Reform Bill 2006 Paragraph 42(1))*

Section 10(2) Coroners Act 1988 covers the Coroner's powers to deal with failure to attend or failure to give evidence.

When faced with a witness declining to give evidence, the CI needs to be able to explain not only the above, but also that in fact the giving of a statement can be advantageous to that person. A statement is a guide to the Coroner as to what that person does or does not know. With it the Coroner can ascertain whether or not that person needs to attend, and what areas the Coroner will want to ask about. Without such information the Coroner is going to have to bring the witness to court, in case they have valuable information, and will have to ask them about everything possible – thus lengthening the person's time in the witness box. Such explanation usually overcomes the misunderstanding and the statement is forthcoming.

13.08 Witness is far away

Sometimes it is not practicable to meet a witness face to face. The witness may live far away or overseas. They may not want to travel to the place where the person died. (This is not unusual, even with partners or parents - some do want to visit the exact place of death and lay flowers for example. Many do not want to visit the town or even country that has unwittingly been involved in their grief.) Possible resolutions are:

13.08.1 Technology

E-mails, faxes and telephone conversations, are all acceptable ways of communicating with such individuals.

13.08.1.1 E-mails

E-mails are especially useful with relatives, family or witnesses living abroad where time differences could potentially cause problems. E-mails have the advantage of being retainable both electronically as well as in hard copy. Copies can be printed off for the Coroner to show the communication efforts that have been made. They can be kept on the file for the future, should a relative later claim that efforts to trace them were not made.

E-mailed statements cannot be signed but this is not a problem for the Coroner as there is no legal requirement that information must be signed and dated even though it is preferable, as already discussed above.

13.08.1.2 Faxes

Faxes are similarly useful - although with increasing technology worldwide more people have access to computers (especially at home) than they do to faxes.

13.08.1.3 Telephones

Telephone is still the primary means of communicating with friends, family and witnesses.

There is not a problem with obtaining a statement from someone by interviewing the witness over the telephone. If this is done there are certain basic steps:

- Make notes of what is said (retain the original notes on the file)
- Type it into a statement format
- Send it through the post with a covering letter advising the maker that it is their statement, that they can amend, alter or add as they wish, then sign it and return it and the amendments will be made before the statement goes with the rest of the file to the Coroner
- Ask them to include any documentary exhibits that have been mentioned
- Enclose a reply paid envelope

A sample covering letter is included at Appendix 5.

It is of course important to consider the wishes of the witness as far as possible while consistent with the needs of the Coroner's inquest system.

In some instances witnesses that are not far away geographically prefer to write their own "statements" for the Coroner. They may feel it easier to take their time, write what they wish, rewrite it until it reads as they want. In such circumstances there is a risk that the information the Coroner needs will not be included. It is possible to avoid this by advising in a letter what they should include. Their response can be in a letter and does not need to be on a statement form.

A sample information request letter is included at Appendix 6.

13.08.2 Intermediary

Another means of obtaining evidence from a far off witness is to ask another person to obtain the statement. This can have its difficulties - as discussed above under section 13.3 above.

13.09 Reservations, problems and resolution strategies

There will sometimes be individuals who have reservations about providing information let alone putting it down in statement form. How then can a CI deal with such cases? Some possible blocks and resolution are suggested below.

13.09.1 Don't trust officials

Find out what the block is. If it is a bad experience in the past from an official, stress that you are not there to cause them difficulty, embarrassment or get them into trouble - or whatever it was that gave them the negative reaction. Explain the difference in this situation. A way of gaining trust is to acknowledge that yes, this is a bureaucratic system - they know that anyway. If it is denied then the mistrust will deepen. However for all its bureaucracy - the coronial system is also about speaking for the dead and not letting truth be hidden. The COA motto reflects this: "Advocates for the dead to safeguard the living".

13.09.2 Don't want to "speak ill of the dead"

This may be where the perception is that talking about the deceased's mental condition, suicidal thoughts, financial situation, criminal activity, marital relationships etc. may be "speaking ill of the dead". Here the CI needs to be able to reassure the witness that unless such information is relevant to the circumstances surrounding the death, the Coroner will not raise it in court. However, it is difficult for the Coroner to know what can be avoided – if the information is not available in the first place. Additionally the witness can be advised that one outcome of the Coroner's inquest is to allay rumour and gossip.

13.09.3 Concern about incriminating oneself

The CI should reassure the witness that they are not there to gather information about them - but about the deceased. It is possible to write down that the deceased used drugs - without writing that the statement maker used drugs. The Coroner is not a prosecuting agency and is independent of the police. Coroners are not about judging the activities of the still living and neither are their officers.

13.09.4 Concern about incriminating others

The witness can be advised that information can be given about matters relating to the deceased without naming other individuals. The witness needs to be reassured as to the purposes of the Coroner's inquest and that it is not there to elicit information about other matters – including other potential crimes.

13.09.5 Irritation

That they have already spoken to some other agency - police, HSE, AAIB, RAIB etc – and / or even their employer for an internal enquiry (e.g. NHS Trust or Prison Service). Multiplicity has already been discussed at section 6.01.3 above.

The CI will acknowledge that it is annoying to go over the same ground again. It can also be extremely distressing. See if the other agency will supply a copy of the information already supplied - check that it contains all the information the Coroner's investigation needs. If not - what extra is needed? Restrict the additional statement to these extras only. This will reduce the impact on the statement maker.

If however it is not possible for some reason to access the previously supplied information, stress the importance of this independent investigation. Again stress the ethos of respecting the deceased by such a thorough independent investigation. Explain the Coroner service is not there for prosecution but to establish the facts.

13.09.6 Misunderstanding (of what a witness is in a Coroner's investigation)

"I can't be a witness: I did not see anything; I don't know anything; I was not there when x died."

Explain that a witness is anyone who has relevant information about the deceased - relevant being determined by the Coroner. It is not until the information is obtained that it is possible to tell whether they can help or not. It is therefore important to record what they have to say.

13.09.7 Embarrassment

Embarrassment may be at having a different perspective about the deceased - perhaps from others - especially a partner or parent.

The CI will discuss that our friends see a different side of us than our partner or parent - and that it was no different for the deceased. It is natural that different witnesses have different perspectives. The coronial system is also about speaking for the dead and not letting truth be hidden.

13.09.8 Don't want to be involved

Point out to them that they are already involved. If necessary, just talk to them without writing anything down. Once you have got the information you need tell them that they have told you what is needed and all you need to do is write it down, check it with them to ensure you have understood correctly and get them to sign it

13.09.9 Don't want to have to go to court

Establish what the concern is. It may be fear – of the unknown, of intimidation; it may be that they are disabled or there is some physical difficulty in actually getting to court; perhaps there are emotional and psychiatric problems and the simple act of attendance will make them seriously unwell. The CI can explain that they will not necessarily have to go to court just because they give a statement. They can be advised that their concerns will be put to the Coroner who will consider whether their attendance in person is necessary given the circumstances. See Coroners Rules 1984 rule 37 regarding the use of documentary evidence in the inquest. Under the Coroners and Justice Bill Schedule 4 the Coroner has the discretion to decide which witnesses must appear before him at an inquest hearing. The CI can also offer the witness the opportunity of visiting the court building to see a preceding inquest to see how the Coroner asks questions and what the court layout is.

13.09.10 Child or vulnerable witnesses

There can be very real difficulties in expecting a younger child or a vulnerable witness to give evidence in an inquest. Many Coroners will prefer to deal with such evidence another way. The simplest is to call the person who obtained the statement or information to come to the inquest and present the evidence as hearsay evidence. Thus an officer from the Child Protection team of the local police force may have interviewed a child, established the understanding of the concept of truth, recorded the conversation and had it transcribed, and present the transcription in court, themselves taking the oath in the inquest.

13.09.11 Have been there before

Sadly witnesses may have previously been involved in an inquest and found it to be a "bad experience" or a "waste of time".

13.09.11.1 "Bad experience"

Showing that the CI cares about this witness, asking what made it a bad experience and if possible reassuring them that the same will not happen again should all help overcome a past "bad experience".

- If there is a different Coroner with different ways – explain
- Perhaps the venue will be different – explain
- Perhaps the circumstances of the deaths are completely different

13.09.11.2 "Waste of time"

Explore what made it appear to have been a waste of time. If circumstances are different and there is a likely or possible different outcome, explain. Sometimes a witness cannot be persuaded that an inquest is not a "waste of time". "Exploring Inquests" (op cit) has explored in depth the perceptions of individuals about inquests and their purposes. Experienced CIs will have come across the same reactions in some of the people they have interacted with.

In Chapter 1 some reasons for inquests were outlined and CIs may find it useful to have these observations available.

In a discussion with a well reasoning individual, a CI may find themselves having to agree that in some cases the "system" seems pointless. There is a last resort of "we don't make the system any more than we make the system of taxes or education, we just live in the country that allows such a system to exist. Accordingly we would like your co-operation please". It is not a defeat so much as an acknowledgment that one cannot please all the people all the time. It usually works and witnesses are known to acknowledge the CI's approach to the whole matter, come the inquest itself.

13.10 What if a statement cannot be obtained?

13.10.1 Some people will simply refuse to make a statement
Whatever information they have passed on verbally can be recorded in a statement made by the CI, acknowledging that it is "hearsay". Thus as an example:

"About 1500 on Thursday 5th July 2003 I spoke on the telephone to a Mr J who told me he had known the deceased (Ms F) for about 6 months. He told me he had last spoken to her on the telephone at 1703 on Wednesday 4th July 2003. Mr J informed me that she had said "I am standing on the cliff edge and I am jumping now." Mr J said he had heard the mobile telephone fall to the ground and heard a shout, 'as if of triumph' for a short second. Mr J said he kept the line open and shouted her name down the line. After what seemed like an age but was only 75 seconds according to his mobile telephone, a strange voice spoke on the telephone and told him that someone had just jumped over the cliff.
Mr J informed me that he was not willing to make a written statement and would not sign anything and would not attend court. He declined to give me his address. I made short contemporaneous notes of the conversation at the time in my investigator's notebook number 1235 from which I have written this statement. I produce the original notes as my exhibit CI/1."

Chapter 17 considers the issue of investigator's notebooks in more depth.

13.10.2 Statement never returned signed
Where a "telephone statement" is taken with the witness's knowledge and the draft is sent out with a covering letter and reply paid envelope, there will be occasions when it is not returned. The CI can telephone the witness again and

establish if there was a particular problem (or if it has simply got lost in the post and needs sending again).

The National Crime Faculty published "A Practical Guide to Investigative Interviewing" in 2000 which has since been updated and is obtainable through ACPO. The PEACE framework is expounded in this guide. PEACE stands for Preparation and Planning; Engage and Explain; Account; Clarification and Challenge; Closure; Evaluation. This training is intended for police officers but contains many principles that are applicable to any interviewing. Thus it is worth reading by CIs and the relevant bits extracting.

Gloucestershire Constabulary have placed their policy "Investigative Interviewing Policy" (2007) on their website and it is available to download from www.gloucestershire.police.uk.

There is also a document on this interviewing technique available to download via the UK Border Agency website www.bia.homeoffice.gov.uk policy and law section

14

IDENTIFICATION ISSUES

14.01 Introduction

Identification is always important - not least for the family. In some deaths however the issue of identification is more crucial for the Coroner than in others. In all inquest cases the Coroner needs to know who has died. It is one of the four essentials of the inquest process – who?, where?, when? and how? – as required under Coroners Act 1988 section 11; see also the Coroners and Justice Bill paragraph 5. Under the Coroners and Justice Bill Schedule 4 the Coroner has the discretion to decide which witnesses must appear before him at an inquest hearing. Accordingly CIs may find themselves investing a lot of energy and using all their investigative skills in inquestable deaths to establish the identity of the deceased.

Identification methods can be categorised into:

● Primary – where only one is required   e.g. fingerprints/DNA/implants with unique reference numbers
● Secondary – where two or three are required – including   jewellery/personal effects/distinctive clothing/marks and scars/x-rays showing healed fractures / physical disease (e.g. tumour) and blood grouping
● Supplementary – where primary or secondary is established and these are purely supportive – e.g. visual/photographs/body location descriptions

14.02 Assumptions

In many cases, identification is not too difficult. However assumptions can never be safely made. One scenario where assumptions are likely to be made would be following a road traffic collision. Where the vehicle's Registered Owner is the same gender as the deceased driver it is easy to assume that the two are one and the same. Another occasion when such a mistake can readily be made is where there is a sole occupant of a residence, no signs of forced entry and a deceased of the appropriate gender within the dwelling.

The way to avoid such mistakes is simple – assume nothing, prove everything. The best possible evidence is 100%.

14.03 Different identification approaches

The approach to the identification will vary according to the initial information available. When the probable identity is known, initial efforts are to support or disprove that possibility. Even if it is not the person first considered possible, the chances are that there will be a clear link leading to the correct identification without the need for detailed investigation. Only if and when the first approach falters will the more detailed and complex approach need to be adopted.

14.03.1 Some certainty

When the probable identity of the deceased is known this involves obtaining further evidence to confirm it. For example:

There is a single vehicle RTC; the driver is male; a check of the Police National Computer (PNC) shows the Registered Owner of the vehicle to be a male.

Photographic driving licence or identity card at the scene for instant comparison should be an acceptable level of proof of identity, preferably backed up by formal viewing if the family feel able to, or dental identification if not. The level of acceptability of proof will vary from each Coroner to another and from case to case.

The other time that the identity is known with some certainty tends to be when there is a sole occupant of a residence, there are no signs of forced entry and a deceased of the appropriate gender is found within the dwelling. Again, the best evidence for the Coroner is positive identification – visual or dental. Only if the primary methods fail – as can and does happen on occasion should the Coroner be asked to consider accepting a level of proof of "probability".

Where there is a probable level of identity dental techniques (see section 14.05.3.1 below) can be used as well as DNA (see section 14.05.1 below).

14.03.2 No certainty

The more challenging cases are those where there is no idea of the identity of the deceased. There is nothing about the location of the death to give a clue, and no documentary evidence on the body itself. These are the cases such as a body on the beach; a jumper from a cliff; some suicides. It is cases such as these to whom the rest of this chapter is devoted. How to move from the worst possible scenario with no clues, to the best outcome: positive identification.

14.04 Basic techniques

With any unidentified body, there are certain basics that need recording and certain information that needs capturing as early as possible. It is not always necessary and hopefully only in the extreme cases will the CI stand in the witness box at an inquest and account to the Coroner for all the enquiries made to attempt to identify someone.

It should be noted that it is not failure on behalf of the CI if the deceased with no clues cannot be identified and an "assisted burial" is eventually arranged for an unidentified body. If someone chooses to live and die in such a way that no-one reports them missing or notices that they have disappeared, that is their choice. Ultimately – the coronial system acknowledges that choice.

However it should be borne in mind that it is not just to the Coroner that the CI is accountable – but to the deceased person and their relatives – who may enquire many years later about a case.

14.04.1 Basic physical information to be recorded

Attribute	Specifics and problems
Height	Potential problem: foreshortening due to impact; note that a 'lying down' measurement is recognised as being less accurate than a 'standing up' height
Size	Potential problem: bloating and decomposition may distort the image
Hair (head) colour, length style	Potential problems: hair (and head) may be missing completely; hair may have been dyed, permed or cut after last being seen alive by the informant
Hair (body)	Unshaven armpits? body shaving evidence? Very hirsute parts of torso? Note the body hair colour especially if it is different, or if there is no head hair
Eye colour	Potential problem: the iris loses colour so not always possible to tell; eyes may be missing; there may be false eyes or contact lenses
Teeth	Potential problems: few or no teeth; younger people go to dentist less so fewer people have dental work for charting comparison; no known dentist for comparison
Dentures	Specific: look for evidence of smooth gums
Nail biting	Specific: did they or did they not? People very unlikely to change their habits immediately prior to death
Nail varnish	Specific: was there any? People very unlikely to change their habits immediately prior to death

Piercing holes	Potential problem: may not have jewellery in Specific: still need to chart how many holes and where
Marks, scars, tattoos	Potential problem: when a body is badly decomposed it is not always possible to see a scar or a tattoo even if it is suspected that one was there from other information; skin slippage also distorts marks etc; there may be new blemishes since the informant last saw the deceased; the informant may not have been intimate enough to know about all the marks present (although they may not accept that reality)
Deformities	Potential problem: limbs may be missing because of the circumstances of death or the effects of other elements (e.g. sea) on the body after death Specific: missing limb; cleft palate
Gender signs	Specific: look for external genitalia and be aware of need to check for more than one set, or absence (e.g. in endocrine diseases or transgender scenarios)
Operations	Specific: look for existing additional evidence such as pins; plates Look for absence such as missing areas of anatomy e.g. foreskin after circumcision (but beware if there has been a partial circumcision e.g. due to a phimosis in youth, and the foreskin has grown back. The male may be recorded as having had a circumcision yet the foreskin is present)

The CI quickly learns to be wary of physical information recorded e.g. on missing person forms. This is especially the case where the information was not a parent or relation. A recorded height, for example, may be significantly incorrect and therefore mislead the unwary CI, as can hair colour, as both of these are subjective to the person describing).

All these features go to build up a description of the deceased for circulation – see sections 14.04.5 and 14.04.6 below.

The Police National Computer (PNC) can be searched for significant marks and scars and tattoos. Such searches are of course dependent on the information input by the police when the person was previously detained for example. Thus, information such as "tattoo left arm" is not overly helpful. Contrarily, information such as 'midline abdominal scar 12" long from previous operation' may be very helpful in establishing a deceased's identification.

See also Appendix 7 for a height and weight conversion chart for metric and imperial measures and international clothing sizes

14.04.2 Property

Full details of all property should be recorded. Other than in exceptional circumstances e.g. extreme decomposition, it should not be thrown away. It should be cleaned as thoroughly as possible, recorded, photographed and described.

Destruction should rarely take place and only so long as all are completely satisfied that there is nothing "suspicious" about the matter.

Property	Specifics and problems
Clothing	Labels: check whether the writing is in English or another language, whether the sizing is in English or foreign first; check colour/make/pockets/zips etc
Money	What currency?
Jewellery	Describe; take to jewellers to see if unusual and traceable; look for serial numbers and inscriptions

Other items   Look carefully for information such as labels on rucksacks; security codes or locksmiths' details on keys

14.04.3 Photographs

Photographs should be taken of the body from all angles with special attention to scars, marks, distinctive features etc. A digital camera will make for ease at a later stage. However pictures from a 35mm camera can be scanned into the computer if necessary.

Photographs should be taken as soon as possible after finding the body and before any further decomposition sets in. This is particularly important when the body has been in salt water as decomposition is accelerated under these circumstances. Although a deceased's appearance may not be too bad immediately after retrieval, 24 hours later the decomposition may be well advanced.

Reasonable photographs can be used to identify someone once decomposition makes visual identification undesirable if relatives are found later.

Also, it may be that an artist's impression will need to be made. Photographs are vital to this process. Forensic artists ask for photographs to be taken prior to the post mortem examination to ensure as accurate a likeness as possible. They should be taken in the same plane as the part being identified.

If someone has been detained by police a photograph may have been taken. The PNC will show if a photograph is available. Such information may be a useful tool in identification.

Photographs alone may not be enough to satisfy a Coroner as to the identity of a deceased, but taken in conjunction with another identifying feature the overall result may be conclusive.

Photographs should also be taken of the clothing worn. This should be immediately but also once cleaned if to be kept for a period of time. Clothing can assist in identification and it is easier to circulate photographs than the articles themselves. Photographs can be circulated through the media with a description of the deceased at an early stage.

14.04.4 Fingerprints

Fingerprints should be taken from the deceased as soon as possible after recovery if identity is not established early and is likely to be a problem. Even if a person's fingers are badly decomposed attempts should still be made to obtain them. There are techniques available to improve the quality of prints even under extreme circumstances. This might include injecting saline fluid under the skin to plump it out and reduce wrinkles caused by post mortem changes or prolonged immersion in water. Local police fingerprint experts should be consulted to see what techniques are available in that area. With advancing technology, portable electronic fingerprint readers are now available in many areas which could potentially provide an instantaneous identification once the fingerprints are scanned in and sent to the local police PNC bureau.

Once obtained, fingerprints should be sent to the fingerprint bureau of the local police force. If someone has been detained by police in the past, fingerprints should have been taken. Identity can be established through just one print and fingerprint identification is a primary means of identification. The Immigration authorities also maintain a fingerprint database and it is worth contacting them, perhaps through the special branch of the local police force.

Even if there are no matches after the various searches, fingerprints of the deceased should be retained. At some later stage if a possible identity is put forward, it would be possible to obtain 'latent' prints, from a home address or work place or other personal property of such a person, for comparison.

14.04.5 Local circulation

After all clues have been investigated, but no identity has been established, another course of action is to check with the local police force for details of any missing persons who may match the deceased. Such checks should be made regularly to ensure a report is not missed if made after an initial check has been made. If there is no match, it is advisable to wait for 24 – 48 hours before circulating more widely, in case a missing person report is made, perhaps in a different area, after the deceased has been found.

14.04.6 National circulation

If initial early enquiries fail to establish an identification then details of the deceased should be circulated nationally via the PNC and the other organisations (see section 14.05.4 below for further information).

14.05 Advanced techniques

14.05.1 Deoxyribonucleic acid (DNA)

DNA is inherited from biological parents and is unique to each individual apart from identical siblings (any number) who will have identical DNA as the original cell has replicated exactly.

Non-identical siblings of the same biological parents have similar but not identical DNA.

If someone has been detained by police DNA will have been retained under certain circumstances. DNA testing and checking against the national database is now cheaper and quicker than it was in the past. An average time for testing a non-urgent sample may be two weeks. Who pays for the testing (the Coroner or the police) is an issue that will need to be resolved. Once that has been agreed, arrangements need to be made for who will take what samples and how they will be processed through to the Forensic Science Service. Liaison with the Scientific Support Branch of the local police force will ascertain what will be the best samples under the specific circumstances to achieve the required outcome.

DNA degrades over time so that samples of blood, hair and deep thigh muscle taken soon after death may provide sufficient detail for analysis. However as time passes it is advisable to take samples of bone with good bone marrow – e.g. from the femur, or even teeth. In cases of decomposition or burning the bone marrow is usually protected. Processing bone marrow for DNA takes longer and is more expensive than deep muscle, so will normally only be carried out if muscle fails or is not available.

Mitochondrial DNA is found in hair shafts, bones, teeth, faeces and may be useful if the body is badly burned or decomposed and a full DNA profile is not available. Mitochondrial DNA is passed down through the maternal line only. It therefore only contains half the genetic information in comparison with a full DNA profile. It is therefore much harder to provide a DNA profile of statistical reliability and will generally only be useful where there is already a probable identity of the deceased. In such cases the mother or siblings of the believed deceased can also be tested for their mitochondrial DNA, which should match that of the deceased. Conversely, if the mitochondrial DNA of the probable identity person does not match, that will rule out the probable identity.

Once the DNA is profiled it can be tested against the national DNA database which holds many thousands of records. It is possible that fingerprints will not yield a result but DNA will, particularly if the fingerprints were in poor condition due to the state of the body. However it is unlikely.

The Coroner will usually give permission for the deceased's DNA profile to be retained by the Forensic Science Service in case later information comes to light that will assist in the identification. For instance some months later a potential identification may surface. One way of proving or disproving it would be through DNA from the home address, from the parents, or from a spouse and child combination. Positive DNA identification is a primary means of identification.

The CI should ask for a 'bar graph' printout of the profile to be sent through to them to be kept on the file either until identification is made – or failing that, for ever. This should be kept along with the original dental chart, photographs, and original fingerprints. The reason for keeping everything together is common sense. If someone comes along in the future and a possible identification is made, for all the relevant information about the deceased to be with the relevant Coroner is sensible. For it all to be scattered among the different agencies, e.g. police, FSS etc – makes less sense. The Coroner is one of the first ports of call for enquirers seeking a missing person. The national organisations also put enquirers in touch with the relevant Coroner's area.

14.05.2 Other methods

There may be other clues from the body that can be considered. The pathologist can supply information from the post mortem examination which may further assist the CI. Internal examination yields information about past orthopaedic operations such as joint replacement or fracture repairs. All surgical implants have a unique reference number which can be used to trace back to the recipient details. This may require contacting a local orthopaedic surgeon to establish the make of the prosthesis or implant, and then checking with the manufacturer as to which hospital was supplied with that uniquely referenced item. Enquiries can then be made with that hospital who can check their records and ascertain which patient was fitted with the prosthesis / implant. Such information would in all probability be regarded as primary identification.

Skeletal x-rays may show up such prostheses / implants; or old fractures which could well be regarded as secondary identification.

Cardiac pacemakers each have a unique reference number on them and if such a device is found at post mortem, enquiries can be made of the cardiology department at the local Trust. Even if the device were not fitted in that locality, the information recorded within it can be accessed by them. This information would include the name and the date of birth of the person into whose body the device was implanted. However if the device was fitted outside the UK, the trail may be more complex. Each device contains details of the manufacturer and enquiries can be made with that manufacturer to see which hospital the device was supplied to, in which country, and then investigations taken on from there. The devices also have 'memories' which can be interrogated and the ECG can be downloaded and the timeline extracted which can be a useful tool. This information remains (even after the deceased themselves has been cremated as it will have been removed prior to cremation).

14.05.3 Other specialists

Other specialists may be useful in the identification process and these include anthropologists, forensic artists, facial reconstruction experts, forensic odontologist.

14.05.3.1 Forensic odontologists

A forensic odontologist will be able to compare ante mortem dental charting if supplied by a dentist, with the post mortem evidence they examine. If ante mortem evidence is available a positive identification can usually be made. They can comment on post-mortem loss of teeth; the cavities and decay present.

If there is no ante mortem evidence, the odontologist can still supply useful information which may assist in determining details of the deceased such as the age of a body - by the amount of deciduous and permanent teeth present or partially erupted and the staging of wisdom teeth and their root structure. Similarly they can comment on the likely ethnicity – due to the shape of teeth. This may be helpful in a badly decomposed individual. While this may not initially provide a positive identification, it can assist when a probable identification is made which needs confirmation or otherwise.

The British Association of Forensic Odontologists website www.bafo.org.uk has a guide to forensic odontology on which is stated:

"Forensic odontology is a branch of forensic medicine and, in the interests of justice, deals with the proper examination, handling and presentation of dental evidence in a court of law. The work of a forensic odontologist covers:

- *Identification of unknown human remains through dental records and assisting at the scene of a mass disaster*
- *Age estimations of both living and deceased persons including neo-natal remains*

Unidentified bodies come to light frequently, having drowned, burned, been murdered, having committed suicide or died from natural causes. Usually sufficient evidence is apparent to be able to positively identify the body, but from time to time, this identification will rely on dental evidence. All mouths are different and the trained eye of the forensic odontologist will be able to offer a considerable amount of useful information. Most obvious will be to provide an accurate charting of the teeth and fillings present to compare with dental records of missing persons. This often leads to a positive identification.

Despite recent advances in DNA technology, dental identification still offers a rapid and cost effective approach.

Even if only a few teeth are available, an opinion can still be offered on age, habits, oral hygiene, and individual features which may match with ante-mortem records. Where the subject has no teeth, useful information can still be gleaned from the study of any dentures and by X-raying the jaws and skull.

It is important that the services of a forensic odontologist be sought early in these cases, as much time consuming police work can be avoided given a dental report early in the investigation." (www.bafo.org.uk)

If someone's identity is possibly known, enquiries can be made with the NHS Business Service Authority Dental Services Division (NHS BSA DSD), based in East Sussex. Records are kept there of charges for dental work on anyone registered with an NHS dentist. On receipt of appropriate authority they can provide details of the last known dentist for an NHS dental patient, who can then be contacted and the dental records obtained. Those records can be used by the forensic odontologist for comparison against the deceased.

14.05.3.2 Forensic anthropologists

A forensic anthropologist is able to advise on gender and probable racial background of a deceased and uncover any evidence of pre-existing illnesses (such as rickets or scurvy) that an individual had had before death. They can give evidence as to the height o the individual and may uncover evidence of skeletal abnormalities, such as fused spinal vertebrae or an asymmetrical cranial vault. These factors may assist in identification once a probable identity is known, through comparison against medical records. Using all their training and experience in their specialised field, they may be able to detect past fractures in bones that even a forensic pathologist might not identify. Such fractures may eliminate certain 'possible' identities and provide clues as to other possible identities.

14.05.3.3 Forensic archaeologists

A forensic archaeologist can firstly advise whether bones found are human or not. Once established as human bones and therefore of potential interest to the Coroner and CI, the next important factor is the age of the bones – how long have they been there? If they are from an old burial site which has been disturbed during excavation for example, then the Coroner is not concerned over matters of jurisdiction. It is only once the archaeologist advises that the bones are recent and human that they will become of interest to the Coroner and thus to the CI.

Initially it is very likely that the police will be involved to ascertain whether there is any "suspicion" attached (See Chapter 1). The involvement of the forensic archaeologist from that point on will vary according to the presence or absence of "suspicion" and at what stage that is established.

The information that the archaeologist can supply to help police and coroner includes:

● How long has the body been in that place?

They consider the seasonal detritus such as leaf fall and the absence or presence of root growth through the bones. The more root growth and plant infiltration the longer the bones have been in that place.

● How far have the bones been scattered?

Bones can be disrupted for any number of reasons including earth movements, mechanical interference and animal predation. Archaeologists are often able to use plotting techniques to advise the original locus of the entire body before sections have been moved.

- When a "grave" or concealment place was dug

Soil excavation techniques can ascertain whether a "grave" was prepared in advance and then re-visited at a later stage and the body placed in it. The presence or absence of leaf litter in a "grave" can assist in indicating what time of year the "grave" was dug.

- The manner in which a "grave" or concealment place was dug

By exposing the mechanical marks that are left when a "grave" is dug, the forensic archaeologist is able to indicate the type of instrument(s) used (e.g. spade, digger) and can even indicate whether the "grave" was dug hurriedly, more haphazardly, perhaps in a frenzied manner; or whether it was carefully and more methodically prepared.

14.05.3.4 Forensic entomologists
Following death insects arrive at a body in an order of succession. Thus it is possible for a forensic entomologist to be fairly accurate as to when a death occurred, from the insect evidence available.

14.05.3.3 Forensic palynologists
Palynologists study pollen and grains produced by flowering plants and cone bearing plants and spores produced by ferns, mosses algae and fungi and have extensive knowledge of pollen characteristics. Pollen is seasonally sensitive and occurs in known geographical clusters. The evidence supplied by a forensic palynologist rarely provides conclusive evidence but can provide supporting or non-supporting evidence which can assist in where a body has been prior to being found, and how long a body has been in situ where it is found.

In a case where a number of different "ologists" assist with a death, care has to be taken to ensure that one "ologist" does not interfere with or destroy evidence through their actions, that another "ologist" might have needed. It is likely that such cases will arise when the police have a significant role in the investigation, e.g. in a case of a suspicious death. Thus the issue of which "ologist" attends, and in which order they retrieve the evidence, is usually a strategy decision for an SIO in conjunction with a senior forensic officer.

14.05.4 Other organisations

14.05.4.1 National Policing Improvement Agency (NPIA) Missing Persons Bureau (MPB)

As of 1 April 2008 the National Policing Improvement Agency (NPIA) Missing Persons Bureau (MPB) is based at Bramshill in Hampshire. The front page of their website www.npia.police.uk states:

"The NPIA Missing Persons Bureau (MPB) works alongside the police and related organisations to improve the services provided to missing persons investigations and increase effectiveness.

We act as the centre for the exchange of information connected with the search for missing persons nationally and internationally. The unit focuses on cross matching missing persons with unidentified persons/bodies. Other key activities include:

● *Maintaining records of missing persons and unidentified persons/bodies to provide an investigative support service to police*

● *Maintaining a dental index of ante-mortem chartings of long term missing persons and post-mortem chartings from unidentified bodies"*

(www.npia.police.uk)

On the website there are different sections, eg for police, public and Coroners office

The NPIA MPB publishes a quarterly newsletter "The Bureau" which is available to download from their website www.npia.police.uk

In the September 2008 issue of "The Bureau" it states:

"Our objectives
The Bureau focuses on cross-matching missing persons with unidentified persons/bodies, with the aim of getting a positive match result. We maintain a database of:
● *All persons missing in the UK for over 14 days, or sooner where the force feels the case warrants more urgent attention*
● *All foreign nationals reported missing in the UK*
● *All UK nationals reported missing abroad*
● *All unidentified bodies or persons found within the UK*
We use this database to help match unidentified bodies/ persons to reports of missing persons.
What else do we do?
● *Maintain a dental index of ante-mortem chartings of long term missing persons and post-mortem chartings from unidentified bodies"*

In the April 2009 issue of "The Bureau" it states:

"Our plans for the future include work in a variety of areas, including:
● *The production of new, full guidance on the management, recording and investigation of Missing Persons*
● *International co-ordination building a network of contacts with overseas missing persons bureaux*

The NPIA records details of persons reported missing by police forces and can pass information on to CIs when an unidentified body is found.

On the NPIA website in the police section there are a number of forms including one for reporting details of a found unidentified body – which CIs will be able to use to inform the NPIA MPB of any such bodies in their area.

There is 2005 ACPO guidance on the management and recording and investigation of missing persons (2005). This is not available to download from the ACPO website but is available to download as a pdf from the NPIA MPB website www.npia.police.uk

14.05.4.2 Missing People

The National Missing Persons Helpline rebranded in July 2007 and is now called Missing People. According to their website, this is

"the UK's only charity that works with young runaways, missing and unidentified people, their families and others who care for them " (www.missingpeople.org.uk)

They work closely with the NPIA MPB, but their database has historically been wider than the police's and so possibly more comprehensive. However, from February 2009 Missing Persons no longer works to resolve cases of unidentified people. This means that they no longer register unidentified cases and will only undertake database searches at the request of NPIA MPB. See their website at www.missingpeople.org.uk

14.06 Record keeping of unidentified bodies

All information relating to the body should be retained together in one central place. This would include (non-exhaustive):

- Clothing – which should be laundered to ensure it does not rot
- Property – which may need to be cleaned – to avoid damage – once all possible material has been obtained from it if necessary
- Original fingerprints
- Printout of the DNA code
- Original dental chart
- Photographs
- Artist's impressions
- All documentation including posters for circulation etc; police statements; finder's and any other statements; post-mortem examination and toxicological reports

15

THE CORONER'S INVESTIGATOR - OTHER ROLES

15.01 Introduction

As discussed in Chapter 1 the role of the CI can differ dramatically nationally. Aspects of each role can and do spill into another role. The Coroner and the employer both have some input into what exactly each person in the working environment does.

15.02 CI administrator

This role involves office-based work. Many of the tasks are closely related to secretarial tasks, but require an understanding and familiarity with the underlying procedures. In some areas Coroners may have administrative assistants who perform some or all of these functions. The tasks are likely to include amongst others:

- Passing of sudden death forms to the pathologist
- Preparation of forms for the Registrar of Births and Deaths (currently: forms 100A, 100B, 99, 120 and 121)
- Distributing leaflets and forms to relatives
- Preparation of disposal forms including Certificate A and Cremation Form 6
- Preparation of interim death certificates in an inquest case
- Informing GPs of the cause of death after a post mortem
- Cataloguing and storage of evidence
- Returning of property not required as evidence, to the appropriate family member/executor, if not done by the police
- Arranging the processing and binding of photographs

- Putting together the Coroner's file for an inquest
- Fixing a date for the inquest
- Booking the court venue, date and time
- Sending out the witness notices and / or summons
- Preparing accurate witness list for the court
- Ensuring adequate copies of evidence for Coroner and witnesses
- Arranging the audio recording of inquests and storage or transcription of the tapes themselves
- Arranging a jury
- Sending out juror summons and accompanying paperwork
- Arranging return of evidence / property / notes etc. after the inquest
- Filing of paperwork

15.03 CI family liaison

This role may be undertaken both in the office and outside. It involves dealing with the family, executors, solicitors or other significant people; explaining the role of the Coroner; the need for any post mortem, and advising on representation at a post mortem or inquest.

The government's position paper (2004) notes that:

"Coroners' officers would need to continue to maintain close links with bereaved families throughout the death investigation process." (op cit paragraph 60)

The work may include:

- Explaining the time scales involved to family/friends
- Informing the family or other significant persons of the cause of death, whether organs/tissues have been retained and what options may be available
- Informing the family about the Certificate A process if appropriate and establishing their views on the doctor issuing a medical certificate
- Answering any questions the family may have and giving them contact numbers for other agencies

- Explaining about the registration arrangements in the area
- Providing information on funeral directors in the area

This role can be emotionally very demanding and time consuming depending on the particular circumstances of the case and the people involved. However it can also be the most rewarding aspect of a CI's role.

15.03.1 Cause of death

The cause of death is given by pathologists in medical terminology. Lay people may not always understand the terminology. An important aspect of this role for any CI is to "translate" the medical words into words the individual can accept and understand.

It is always wise to ask the person how much medical knowledge they have before starting such an explanatory translation – to avoid the embarrassment of explaining to a surgeon for example what a ruptured aneurysm is!

Once that fact is established, an offer to explain the medical terms into "lay person's English" can be made. Such translation should always be given with the proviso that the CI is not a doctor and that the other person can always ask a doctor to translate it all more precisely if they wish.

Often what relatives need at this stage is a ready phrase to tell all the family and friends who are asking why the person has died. Thus "it was a heart attack" or "his heart just wore out" or "his arteries were all clogged up" may well be all that is needed, even if not medical.

This stage of a CI's work involves a judgment call as to how much information the person on the other end of the telephone wants and needs and can cope with. Such judgment calls are made on very little information and it is important to be sensitive to the other person. Checking by asking "are you all right with that?" or "does that make sense?" is advisable. Allowing the recipient of the information to read back the information provided or ask any questions is helpful.

In some instances people want more information and the CI may need an in-depth knowledge of what an aneurysm is, how it forms, why it was not spotted or treated etc. However, it is important for CIs to know the limitations of their own medical knowledge and not to embroider or state anything they do not know. Relatives will often take the description as "gospel" and if they later find it to be wrong – will let the CI know in no uncertain terms. Thus if CI find themselves out of their depth – the person should be advised that they will need to consult their own GP – or the deceased's GP if different. Sometimes they can be referred to the pathologist themselves.

15.03.2 Death registration

This involves informing the family how and where to register the death and what other paperwork is available from the Registrar of Births, Deaths and Marriages.

15.03.3 Tissue and / or organ retention

(For ease, tissue will be taken in this paragraph to include organs)

Under the Coroners (Amendment) Rules 2005, if a pathologist needs to retain tissue to assist with his investigations on behalf of the Coroner, he has to advise the Coroner who then authorises (or not) the retention of the tissue. If tissue is retained the family have the right to know that it has been retained, exactly what has been retained, and how long the Coroner has authorised the retention to continue. The family then have the right to decide what should happen to the tissue once the Coroner's authority has ceased. The family may choose to delay the funeral of the deceased until the tissue is returned to the deceased's body.

It is apparent therefore that the CI will need to have the skills to explain all this to the family in understandable language and to ensure that the family's wishes are known. Different Coroner's areas have different audit trails for the recording of the facts of such conversations and of the relatives' wishes.

15.03.4 Inquest procedures

This involves explaining why there is to be an inquest, explaining the process, discussing the timing of key events, explaining about obtaining information or evidence, helping the family at the inquest, and providing continuity.

15.03.5 Return of property

This involves explaining about the return of possessions or property or clothing to the appropriate "next of kin" but also about the return of evidence when appropriate in an inquest case.

15.04 CI public relations

As the role of CI becomes better known so demands to liaise with outside agencies increase. Audiences for an explanation of the role include St John Ambulance; different religions and religious sects; GPs and hospital doctors. An input to the various police practitioners is increasingly important. The Coroner's Office has to liaise with the media on a regular basis.

The government's position paper (2004) sees a place for public relations:

"In accordance with recommendations from the Fundamental Review and the Shipman Inquiry, we aim to raise the public profile (sic) of the service. We propose to do this by encouraging coroners to initiate or to continue programmes of public events, including visits and talks, in order that the public has a better understanding of their work." (op cit paragraph 27)

This does not necessarily mean that the Coroners will be the front speakers themselves – it leaves this open. It is possible that the CI will find this aspect of their current role increasing with the overall increase in publicity for the Coroner's service.

15.05 CI court usher

This role always involves attendance at the court, and may include:

- Meeting the witnesses and family
- Managing any tensions between witnesses and family members
- Ensuring all expected witnesses are present
- Explaining the layout of the court, the available facilities, and prohibitions
- Explaining about taking the oath, establishing any particular needs, and ensuring that any particular religious requirements can be met
- Explaining the conduct of the hearing and identifying the people present
- Explaining about the media in and out of the court room, what they are entitled to do and say and what the witnesses and family are entitled to do and say
- If summonsed witnesses not present, calling for them in accordance with statutory requirements so the Coroner can take action against the absent witness, if necessary
- In the courtroom, swearing in the witnesses
- Ensuring all exhibits required for the court that day are available for the Coroner
- Controlling any recording equipment used
- Providing accurate witness list for the media
- Processing fees and allowances for witnesses

In some areas Coroners may have administrative staff who perform many of these functions.

15.05.1 Difficulties with witnesses

The CI can prove invaluable to the Coroner by providing information about any difficulties with witnesses – before the inquest is listed and at the court before it starts.

Should the witness themself die before the inquest is held the Coroner needs to know so that he can advise any advocates as appropriate and inform them of the intention to treat that evidence as documentary evidence under s37 of the Coroners Act 1988.

If there are tensions between different witnesses or between a witness and the family, such as can classically occur at an inquest hearing following a road traffic collision death, the Coroner and their Investigator can develop a strategy to prevent matters degrading into a physical fight in the court on the day.

If there is a feeling that the witness may not attend a summons should be served rather than a notice issued. Even then a witness may disregard the summons and fail to appear on the day. Section 10(2) of the Coroners Act 1988 provides the Coroner with powers to impose a fine (not exceeding £1000). However CIs in their Court Usher role must first "openly call" the witness three times.

15.05.2 Jurors

In an inquest hearing where a jury is required there are additional duties to be performed by either the CI or some other person and these may include in addition to the above:

- Checking that all jurors are present and their details accurate
- Explaining a little about their role and that the Coroner will advise them of their legal duties and responsibilities
- Taking the bailiff's oath regarding the care of jurors
- Establishing any likely conflict that may make a juror unsuitable and liaising with the Coroner
- Processing fees and allowances for jurors

Thomas et al (2002) comment on the importance of this role:

"The coroner's officer therefore provides an important function of the hearing and his or her role should not be overlooked. He or she can provide crucial assistance and information prior to and on the day of the hearing." (op cit 175 – 176)

16

TRAINING

16.01 Introduction

The importance of training is recognised in all disciplines. Employers are recognised as having a duty to train their personnel to perform their role adequately and to equip them with the necessary skills.

Training for CIs has been patchy over the years. It was generally assumed that CIs had the requisite skills by virtue of their having been former police officers. For a large part of the CI's role this may have been the case, although the medical knowledge often still needed to be learned. However as the role of CIs has developed, so the need for further training beyond police knowledge has increased. Similarly as more CIs have no police background, such an attitude is no longer tenable.

Hansard records the debate in the House of Commons on 4/12/2008 that Sir Alan Beith MP stated:

"..funding for coroners, their staff and training needs to be more consistent. If people had not read our report or did not know the system they would be amazed by the extent of its diversity. In some areas, the local authority pays for coroners' offices; in others, the police pay for them; and in others, coroners are serving police officers—an arrangement that is sometimes pragmatically convenient—and there is no real consistency. There is also little consistency about providing and paying for training so that coroners' officers and other staff can fulfil the needs of the families with whom they deal. Some of them do a superb job—indeed, I have

heard much testimony to the quality of the work that some coroner's officers do – but the system is inconsistent and sporadic."
(www.parliament.uk/publications/hansard)

In his introduction to the government's position paper (2004) the Home Secretary stated that:

"The new coronial system we propose must be:
Professional *(sic) – its staff will be better regulated than at present and will benefit from continuous professional development, including training to high standards."*

The government's position paper (2004) continues:

"Currently there is no universal **coroner's officer training**. *(sic) In due course, we would want all officers to receive mandatory training as soon after appointment as practical.* **Support and administrative staff** *(sic) should also have access to relevant training opportunities." (op cit paragraph 62)*

"The Chief Coroner may, with the agreement of the Lord Chancellor, make regulations about the training of ..... coroners' officers and other staff " (Coroners and Justice Bill Paragraph 28)

The previously mentioned MoJ / COA 2008 survey (See section 1.03) also asked questions of Coroner's Officers and Coroner's staff about training.

Following the Queen's speech to Parliament on 3/12/2008 the Coroners' Society of England and Wales (CSEW) issued a press release:

"the Society looks forward to all necessary improvements in infrastructure, Court accommodation, Coroners' officer numbers and coroners' staff training that will be necessary in a service designed for modern times." (www.coronersociety.org.uk)

The Coroners' Society of England and Wales (CSEW) placed a copy of its submission to the Public Scrutiny Committee in February 2009 on its website in which it stated:

"The Society recognises that, given the lack of Treasury investment, the real reform will be non-legislative, the most important part of which will be persuading local authorities to invest in the coronial service infrastructure. Not far behind this would come the development of the role of the Coroner's Officer as a recognised career, with a national training qualification with ongoing professional development." *(para 51)*
(www.coronersociety.org.uk)

The University of Teesside in association with the COA runs a number of modular accredited courses for personnel within the Coroners' service. These include

Coroner's Law and Bereaved course, a two week course described on the COA website:

"A 2 week course with an introduction to Coroner's law, death certification and registration, issues such as religious and cultural perspectives of death, ethical practice, effective communication etc." *(www.coronersofficer.org.uk)*

16.02 Training for CIs and MEOs

Chapter 1 explored how the role of the MEO is fundamental in all deaths. It follows therefore that knowledge of matters medical is vital. In that chapter the point was made that CIs also need to have a good sound medical understanding, an aspect of their role which has been reinforced in subsequent chapters.

Chapter 15 explored how the family liaison role of the CI involves translating medical terminology into a language that families can understand. Before they can do this – they need to understand for themselves. Medical knowledge is therefore crucial as is access to medical dictionary or other literature.

Increasingly more CIs come from a background involving medical knowledge, which gives an advantage. Where they have little or no knowledge however, training should be given.

The University of Teesside in association with the COA runs a two week course for personnel within the Coroners' service and related disciplines: Fundamental Medicine for the Coroner Service. This is described on the COA website:-.

"A two week course dealing with medical terminology, anatomy and physiology, diseases and procedures and their potential complications in the context of sudden death and referral to the Coroner." (www.coronersofficer.org.uk)

16.03 Training for CIs

This should encompass all areas raised in this book but should also specifically include an understanding of:

- Scientific techniques
- Forensic science and toxicology
- Policing functions, including investigation techniques, methods available and legal requirements
- Laws including homicide, corporate manslaughter, assisted suicide, human rights; coronial laws
- Road traffic collisions, investigation, reconstruction, road traffic management and road safety campaigns
- Legal issues surrounding deaths in custody, the role of the police custody officers, prison procedures
- Legal issues surrounding deaths in mental health institutions
- Evidence and the rules of evidence in relation to the Coroner
- The roles and functions of outside agencies in relation to sudden death e.g. Fire Service/HSE/local authorities
- The role in multiple fatalities / major disasters
- Illegal and legal drugs with a knowledge of terms in relation to availability, use, signs symptoms and analysis

It should also include an ability to:

- Assist the role of the scientific support branch officers (including the requirements in relation to property as exhibits, the recording and continuity of samples)
- Attend the post mortem examination when required
- Take photographs

The University of Teesside in association with the COA runs a course: Medico-legal Death Investigation:

"A two week course, looking at effective death investigation on behalf of HM Coroner, it deals with the role of staff gathering information for the Coroner, pathologists and inquests" . (www.coronersofficer.org.uk)

Participation in training on emergency planning by the police or local authorities, whether tabletop, theoretical or practical would be advisable

16.04 Training for CI - statement taker & evidence gatherer

This should encompass everything raised in Chapter 13 of this book and specifically an understanding of:

- The importance of the section 9 CJA paragraph
- The Coroner's options of reading statements if there are no objections from "properly interested persons" so that the statement taker does not always have to go to the inquest
- Confidentiality; ownership; disclosure; copyright issues; data protection issues - the release to and obtaining of documents from varied sources and agencies and application of the Data Protection Act 1998
- The need to explain that the statement will be made available to the police if a death becomes "suspicious"
- The need to explain why the information needs to go into a statement form
- The need to obtain other relevant information that may inform the coroner as to the conduct of his investigation

- The need to obtain documentary evidence and produce this as an exhibit
- The need to obtain exhibits
- The need to bag, tag and label evidence in compliance with police requirements, if required

The training should also ensure that the CI has an ability to conduct effective interviews of witnesses and relatives (face to face and by telephone).

16.05 Training for the CI – administrator

This is essentially the same as for an administrator in any field. An ability to prioritise, organise, be methodical and foresee the consequences of changes to any system are vital. Additionally there is the need to understand the role of the Coroner and the CI.

16.06 Training for the CI - family liaison

This should include:

- Understanding when a post mortem examination will be required and why
- Full knowledge of coronial law including removal of a body out of England & Wales
- Knowledge of organ and tissue retention practice and procedures
- Bereavement counselling skills, to include dealing with grief and knowledge of further options available in counselling
- Time management and stress management skills
- Knowledge of the various support groups, availability and the facilities offered by such organisations as Cruse, Victim Support Services (VSS), Survivors of Bereavement by Suicide (SOBS), Foundation of the Study of Infant Deaths (FSID), INQUEST etc.
- Understanding of the role of the Registrar, and cremation regulations and working practices
- Understanding of arrangements for evidence/possessions/property/ clothing
- Basic knowledge of probate issues and where further information may be obtained
- Understanding of the police FLO role

- Ability to deal fairly and sympathetically with people, of whatever race, colour, ethnic origin or sexual orientation
- Understanding of minority cultural and religious practices and requirements

16.07 Training for CI - court usher role

This should include:

- Public speaking and assertiveness
- Knowledge of powers available to control the court, and relevant offences
- Knowledge of legal consequences for non-attendance by witnesses or jurors
- Arrangements for the production of witnesses by the prison service or police
- Knowledge of layout of court building and location of retiring rooms, facilities, hours of cafeterias etc.
- Understanding of the different religious oaths and requirements, and knowledge of location of appropriate holy books
- Understanding of the rights and limitations in relation to the media
- Understanding of the allowances and fees available for witnesses and jurors
- Knowledge of the 'jury bailiff' role

Annex 3 of the government's position paper (2004) states its intention to provide within three years:

"Improved support for the Coroner's Officers Association training for coroner's officers."

A three year undergraduate degree course has been developed to run at the University of Teesside.

Despite all the available training it is still the case that many CIs are self-taught and therefore to the level of their own interest. Many attend courses in their own time and at their own expense.

17

CORONER'S INVESTIGATORS' EQUIPMENT

17.01 Introduction

It has been demonstrated that the role of CI is complex and demanding.

As dedicated CIs' roles develop, the accountability will increase. This relates to the accountability of each CI – be they medical or forensic or dually experienced. However there is also the accountability of the employer to the Investigator.

With that in mind this chapter considers possibly some of the most important aspects of death investigation – equipment and record keeping.

17.02 Medical record keeping

Each death investigated by the CI needs accurate records. For example:
- What enquiries were made?
- Of whom?
- What decisions were reached?
- By whom?

17.02.1 Standardisation

It may be that standard forms are developed providing national consistency which could include (non exhaustively):

- GP details – name, address, telephone and facsimile numbers
- When the person had last consulted a GP – date?
- Reason for that consultation?

- When last seen by others from medical profession. Who? When? Where? Why?
- Hospital/hospice doctor details
- Investigations that have been carried out with details and results if known
- Diagnosis/differential diagnoses reached
- Can a doctor issue a medical certificate as to cause of death (MCCD)?
- Do the family have information which would cast doubt on the medical opinion such as might cause the Coroner to consider a post mortem examination is necessary?
- Record details of family representative with whom matters were discussed: name, relationship to deceased; address, telephone numbers
- Details of accepting authority – name, position

Currently every CI records different information – as expected of them by their Coroner. This may change with a national system, whether it is imposed through legislation, or developed through best practice procedure.

17.03 Investigative records

17.03.1 Introduction

Record keeping has always been of importance to the police. However, in the light of the report into the Stephen Lawrence Inquiry by Sir William Macpherson of Cluny (1999), and other enquiries since, police increasingly recognised the importance of keeping accurate logs in all major investigations. Training was instituted for SIOs and FLOs in crime and road traffic deaths.

In every such death the investigative process could come under scrutiny. Therefore a policy for dealing with inquestable deaths, and for recording of contacts made, is good practice.

CIs may be called as witnesses to any court. Not just the Coroner's Court as is routinely expected, but also to criminal or civil courts. CIs therefore need to be able to account for their actions, with documentary evidence. Such material may be disclosable and may be sensitive.

The accountability of CIs is already increasing and is likely to increase more in the future – not less.

17.03.2 How does this apply to the CI?

Each employer of a CI will have different methodology and rules about how to keep a log and what to put in it.

There are two main suggested approaches that are already in use in different parts of the country.

17.03.3 A multi-function notebook

In some areas where police are the employer of the CI, "investigator's notebooks" are currently in use. Police CID officers regularly use such notebooks at the scene of a suspicious death. Everything to do with the case is recorded in this notebook at the scene. In the case of the SIO it will also include policy decisions.

The CI can use the "investigator's notebook" for a multitude of purposes. Some are listed below (in no particular order):

17.03.3.1 Time recording

- Time started work each day
- Time finished work each day
- Breaks taken
- Time recalled to work

This is of value to the employer, but also helps the CI when completing time sheets/claim forms.

17.03.3.2 Daily activity log

A notebook can also provide a daily activity record for each day:

- What time the CI left the office to attend the scene of a death or the mortuary or the court for an inquest

- The time of arrival at the relevant location
- The mileage incurred (which can assist in completion of the claim forms at the end of the claim period)
- Overtime incurred – whether for payment in money or time - or not being claimed at all but still needing recording for European Hours Directive etc

17.03.3.3 Description of the deceased

When attending a scene, full details can be recorded in the notebook including description, body, clothing, position (see Appendix 3 for the generic checklist). It may need top be very detailed if photographs are not taken for some reason.

17.3.3.4 Actions taken at the scene

Brief notes can be recorded which will be subsequently be the basis for a full statement. These notes would quite possibly be disclosable under the rules of the Criminal Procedure and Investigations Act 1996 (CPIA).

17.03.3.5 Details of evidence seized

- Full description. How big? How much? How many? What colour?
- What?
- Why seized
- Exact location at the scene in relation to other objects

Details can be transferred on to any official form at a later stage.

17.03.3.6 Details of people spoken to

Names, addresses and telephone numbers can all be obtained from family, witness, other significant people – and of persons not present but considered important

17.03.3.7 Advantages of this system:

- For each individual inquestable death any details can be recorded in this notebook. An entry in the margin can details the name of the deceased – or the case number – for ease of reference at a later date

- The notebook can be carried at all times – giving an easy record at the scene of any death. Details of evidence at the scene, witness details, deceased details, sketch map etc – anything can be recorded at the scene
- Telephone conversations can be resumed at the time being held in the notebook
- The notebook has sequentially numbered pages. This makes it a credible document should it later be needed in another court
- "Tamper proof" - ESDA tests can be applied to it (Electrostatic Detection Apparatus)
- Each notebook is itself uniquely numbered and the issue number can be recorded centrally by an administrator. At the end of one notebook the number of the next one can be recorded and at the start of the next notebook the unique number of the previous notebook can be recorded – again offering a degree of security that the court system appreciates
- Once completed the notebook can be stored safely and retrieved as original notes if required at a later stage
- If the inquestable case is a complex one; or the family demand a great deal of interaction; or it is thought that the inquestable death will be an involved one – such as a prison death – one book can be uniquely allocated to a specific case. The original ongoing book continues to act as previously, but this notebook is specifically for this case. In the main ongoing notebook reference is made with to the book in existence for the particular case and the unique number cross referenced

17.03.3.8 Disadvantages of this system:

- Not every reference to one case is kept with the case papers. This can be frustrating and time consuming if evidence is needed at a later date
- The notebook stays with the CI all the time – and not on the file. Thus, if the CI is out of the office and an enquiry comes in – colleagues cannot access the information in the notebook at the time and have to explain to the caller that the CI concerned will need to call back to deal with the enquiry. However this is not usually a problem. The rapport that a CI builds up with families in inquest cases is such that a delay is not usually an issue

17.03.4 Individual case logs

An alternative system is to have a system of recording information on each inquestable case. More CIs are used to this sort of system. There may be separate sheets for each case for example:

- Description of the deceased, position found and of the entire scene
- Actions taken at the scene
- Details of evidence seized
- People spoken to – a contact sheet

17.03.4.1 Advantages of this system:

- This system allows for separate pre-formatted sheets for each different aspect of the inquestable case. The exact format of these will vary from one Coroner's jurisdiction to another and from one CI to another
- Every reference to one case is kept with the case papers
- If the CI for the case is out of the office and an enquiry comes in – colleagues can access all information relating to that case and can add to it then and there
- All CIs in the same office know where to go on any file to look for the relevant information if they have to answer an enquiry

17.03.4.2 Disadvantages of this system:

- The CI will still need to have some separate recording system for all the bureaucratic requirements of the role
- There will be a number of pieces of paper, which can be scrappy, relating to any death
- There is no telephone conversation log
- Individual pieces of paper are not sequentially numbered pages. They may have less credibility in another court as they could have been written at any time
- Individual pieces of paper are not "tamper proof". ESDA tests cannot be applied

17.03.5 A combination approach

A third option is a combination of the two approaches.

- A notebook is maintained by the CI and contains all details outlined above
- Back in the office the pre-formatted sheets can be kept in the file. The original record from the notebook could be copied or typed onto the file as "scene attendance notes" (for example) so that all colleagues can read them if necessary

When a CI is called to a case where it is immediately apparent from the outset that it will be treated as "suspicious" or that it is going to be a complex case – such as a death in custody – an individual notebook can be used just for that case with cross referencing to the main notebook.

The important thing perhaps is not which system is chosen but the fact that acknowledgment is made that a clear and easily identifiable system is good practice, and if not already in place, should be introduced.

17.03.6 Check lists

A useful tool for CIs, especially in complex enquiries, is a series of checklists and an action plan. A sample action plan is included at Appendix 9. Sample checklists for falls; head injuries; Warfarin treatment; asbestos related deaths are included at Appendices 11, 12, 13 and 14.

17.04 Equipment needed by the CI

The CI needs to be able to attend the scene of any sort of death at any time of any day - from an overdose to a multiple fatality. They need to be fully equipped by their employers with all the equipment to meet employers' responsibilities as regards Health and Safety.

- Mobile phone (with hands free kit for the vehicle)
- Fluorescent jacket e.g. for road traffic collisions/railway deaths/multiple fatalities (if properly marked this also provides easy recognition by emergency service personnel)
- Hard hat e.g. for building sites

- Heat resistant boots and heat resistant gloves e.g. for fire related deaths
- Camera
- Tape measure
- Torch
- Magnifying glass
- Gloves (disposable and needle stick and heat resistant)
- Overshoes
- Protective oversuit
- Warm clothing e.g. hat, fleece jacket, warm gloves
- Evidence bags to collect any items – documentary or otherwise
- Sharps containers and needle resistant gloves - for seizing knives, needles, pointed objects
- Sample bottles - for collecting water at a drowning
- Identity card – the CI should always be able to identify themselves to officials, family, friends, and next of kin

The HOWP Report (2002) considers adequate protection and equipment for Coroner's Officers (op cit Part Three) and makes recommendations along similar lines to those above.

17.05 Psychological equipment

As well as the physical equipment needed, the CI needs to be adequately psychologically supported and protected. It is now well recognised that regular exposure to the grief of others can have an impact on those liaising with the bereaved. Each individual case may only take a small amount of time in the bereaved's situation, but the effect on the CI dealing almost entirely with grieving people is cumulative. Line managers may well have in place regular "debriefing" for their CIs, with counselling or welfare support, and time built into work rosters. The employer's responsibility to ensure the well-being of their staff means that it is not acceptable to assume that CIs can cope or else they would not have taken on the job".

More dynamic may be the impact of traumatic death scenes. The need for critical incident debriefing is recognised by the emergency services such as the police, ambulance, fire service and coastguard. Wherever possible the CI should be involved in any multi-agency debrief, as well as receiving their own.

APPENDIX 1

POLICE HIERARCHY

Police ranks are denoted by the epaulettes worn on police uniforms. Every British police officer is designated his or her own unique number when he joins the service. These numbers are unique within each police force, rather than nationally. So, there may be a PC 538 in Essex and one in Kent. Some forces also show the initial letter of the surname so in Sussex there may be a J538.

The warrant numbers are shown on the epaulettes of Constables and Sergeants only. The warrant number stays with an officer throughout his service within one force, but is not visible on the uniforms above the rank of Sergeant. If an officer moves force, he or she will receive a new warrant number for the new force area.

In all forces, "detective" is a term given to officers who have been assigned to investigative work after completing the appropriate selection and training. Detective ranks parallel uniformed ranks and range from Detective Constable to Detective Chief Superintendent. However it is not usually possible to tell the rank of a detective without looking at the individual warrant, as detectives traditionally wear plain clothes not uniform.

For most forces the rank structure is:

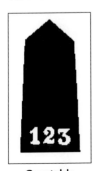 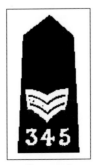 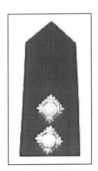

Constable   Sergeant   Inspector

Chief Inspector

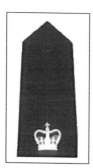

Superintedent

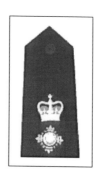

Chief
Superintendent

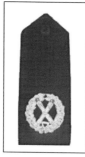

Assistant Chief
Constable

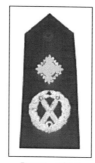

Deputy Chief
Constabl;e

Chief Constable

In the City of London Police the ranks vary above the level of Chief Superintendent:

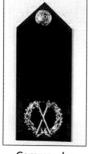

Commander

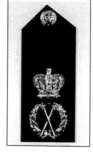

Assistant
Commissioner

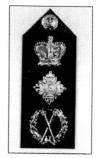

Commissioner

In the Metropolitan Police the ranks vary again for the majority above the rank of Chief Superintendent:

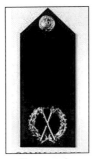

Commander

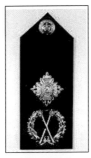

Deputy Assistant
Commissioner

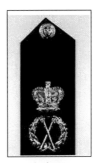

Assitant
Commissioner

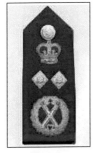

Deputy
Commissioner

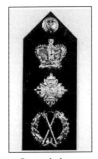

Commissioner

(Information taken from the websites of Essex Police, Metropolitan Police and www.police999.com)

APPENDIX 2

POST MORTEM EXAMINATION

Place:

Date: Time:

DECEASED PERSON'S DETAILS:

Name:

Address:

Date of birth: Place of Birth:

Date died / found dead: Time died / found dead:

Place died / found dead:

Officer identifying to the Pathologist:

PEOPLE PRESENT AT POST MORTEM EXAMINATION:

Pathologist (1): _____

Pathologist (2): _____

Mortuary Technician (1): _____

Mortuary Technician (2): _____

Photographer (1) : _____

Photographer (2): _____

Scenes of Crime Officers: _____

_____

CID Officers: _____

_____

_____

Other Officers: _____

_____

_____

Coroner's Investigator(s): _____

Please forward invoices and post mortem reports to:...

name

Coroner's Investigator

address

Organ Weights		Organ Weights	
Brain		Right lung	
Heart		Left lung	
Liver		Right kidney	
Spleen		Left kidney	
Pancreas			

APPENDIX 3

GENERIC CHECKLIST

A generic checklist that can be applied to all deaths. Specific checklists can also be applied to each individual type of death

The deceased

●	Build of deceased – describe
●	Any known medical condition? Describe, plus its effects on the deceased plus any measures taken to deal with it
●	Is there any relevant mental capacity / incapacity?
●	Is it unusual to find deceased in this place?
●	Had they consumed alcohol immediately prior to incident or shortly before? What? How much?
●	Had they taken any drugs (prescribed or illegal) immediately prior to incident or shortly before? What? How much? By what route?
●	Identification – who is this person? Any means of identification with them? What?
●	Household / living history?
●	Personal details – name, age, date of birth, occupation, social circumstances; GP details

The finder

●	Who is this person?
●	Were they known to the deceased?
●	Were they intimately involved with the deceased?
●	What is their relationship with the deceased?
●	Might the person have been involved in the death and have a part to conceal?
●	What it the finder doing in this place? Is this a regular activity for them? If not – why were they there on this occasion?
●	Date and time found deceased

The body

●	Has the fact of death been verified? Who by?
●	Description of body
●	Are there any wounds on the body that are not consistent with known former injuries or current incident?
●	Are there any signs that the deceased was forced into their current position – bruises on head, arms, wrists, legs, ankles (where restrained)?
●	Is the rigor mortis (limb stiffness) consistent with any account of timing supplied
●	Is the livor mortis (blood pooling) consistent with the history given as to the position in which the body was found? If not why not?
●	Is the position of the body consistent with the history given? If not why not? Was the body moved by the finder for some reason? (not necessarily suspicious)
●	Are there other marks that indicate what may have occurred? e.g. bruises from regularly falling over while drunk; track marks indicative of an IV user
●	Has there been any attempt at resuscitation? By whom? Ambulance personnel or members of public or other?
●	If yes record full details of how many cycles of compression, whether any drugs were administered of so what and in what amounts. Ensure this information is passed to the pathologist prior to post-mortem examination
●	Have any other life-saving measures been carried out eg by ambulance or emergency doctors, such as intravenous cannulation? If yes a record is needed of all attempts at cannulation and marks made on the body through these attempts. This information must be passed to the pathologist prior to post-mortem examination
●	Has any intravenous fluid been given? If so obtain full details of what and how much and pass this information to the pathologist prior to post mortem examination

The scene (where found)

●	Describe fully – indoors, outdoors
●	Temperature – heating on / not, warm / cool time of year
●	Indoors - type of building / storeys / roof / entry points
●	Outdoors - open ground / woods / beach / access routes
●	Health and Safety considerations for all accessing site

Circumstances

●	Aspects of scene particular to the scene – unusual and unexpected findings of scene
●	Aspects of the death particular to the death (these will vary according to hanging, water, electrical etc)
●	Any previous history of address or person(s) involved – e.g. from police or social services

The event

●	Was the event witnessed?
●	By whom?
●	What happened?
●	Is there CCTV footage?

The time

●	Date and time found
●	Were any electrical items on / off?
●	Were the lights on / off?
●	Was the bed slept in / not?
●	Were meals eaten or not – what sort of meal? Did they always have their main cooked meal at lunchtime and it is on the side? Were "Meals on Wheels" delivered? When?
●	The pathologist should be able to give some indication of the nature of last meal (e.g. cornflakes or steak)
●	Were meals eaten or not – what sort of meal? Did they always have their main cooked meal at lunchtime and it is ready to eat on the table? The pathologist should be able to give some indication of the nature of last meal (e.g. cornflakes or steak)
●	Was the deceased wearing day or night clothes?
●	What is the date of the latest newspaper? Are there dated uncollected newspapers in post box? What are their dates?
●	Is there any dated post on the mat or in the box?
●	Are there answerphones on the telephone with a date and time tag? (check to see it is accurate)
●	Is there a TV listings magazine open on a certain date?
●	Are there any lottery tickets – dated? Cashed in for prizes?
●	Is there a calendar ticked off for every day that suddenly stops?
●	Is there a benefits / pensions book with counterfoils of when last collected?
●	Are there any receipts with dates and times?
●	How many dates' worth of benefits / pensions have not been collected?
●	How many days' worth of milk has been left on the doorstep before action was taken?
●	Are there answerphones on the telephone with a date and time tag? (check the actual time showing to see if it is accurate)
●	Mobile telephone – calls or text messages made time / calls or text messages received time / calls or text messages missed time. (Check actual time showing on the device to see if it is accurate)

Other considerations

●	Is there any indication of a suicide note? Where? Is it in deceased's handwriting?
●	Is there any indication of alcohol or drugs paraphernalia or tablet bottles or packets? Where?
●	Is there anything unusual to suggest anything other than a suicide or an accident?
●	Weather conditions over relevant period of time (as best as it is known)
●	Welfare debrief for any involved

Actions

●	Assess safety of scene for yourself and others attending including funeral directors
●	Look for evidence to prove or disprove every possible explanation. Keep an open mind. Assume nothing. Prove everything.
●	Look for suicide note(s)
●	Take photographs
●	Seize any potential evidence - e.g. noose/tablets/syringes/drugs/'sharps containers'/notes/hosepipe/plastic bag/books or other documentary evidence/CCTV
●	Consider internet, emails, text messages, answerphone messages
●	Take measurements. E.g. depth of water/depth of rope above neck/height of deceased/distance to ground/height of building
●	Identification – if not known obtain full descriptive details incl marks scars tattoos/ dental charts/photographs/artist's picture/DNA samples

Statements to be obtained

●	Next of kin – background, identification
●	Finder – with full details in answer to questions outlined in specific section and any other useful information
●	GP – if appropriate; dental practitioner if relevant
●	Psychiatric staff such as consultant, nurses, key workers – if appropriate
●	Any other witnesses as to circumstances, background
●	Any other witnesses covering anything raised above
●	If more than one witness – expect them to differ, record the differences, do not try & persuade them that they have got it wrong and get all accounts to agree
●	Obtain all relevant documentary evidence
●	Download any information relevant to any aspect of the death from the internet

APPENDIX 4

Tablets seized by Coroner's Officer / police in connection with *name of deceased* on date at location

Name	dosage	container	number issued	date issued	tablets remaining	empty blister strips	dosage instructions

Tablets seized by Coroner's Officer Mrs A PERSON in connection with Mr SOMEBODY on 20th February 2003 at 20 Grange Road Anytown

Name	dosage	container	number issued	date issued	tablets remaining	empty blister strips	dosage instructions
Temazepam	5mg	Box	48	19/2/03	2	46	one nocté
co-proxamol	325/32.5	bottle	100	(n/a) OTC	5	n/a	1-2 prn

ALTERNATIVE INFORMATION:
Tablets seized by Coroner's Officer / police in connection with *name of deceased* on date at location

Name	dosage	container	no issued	date issued	issued to whom	tablets remaining	empty blister strips	dosage instructions	location

Tablets seized by Coroner's Officer Mrs A PERSON in connection with Mr SOMEBODY on 20th February 2003 at 20 Grange Road Anytown

Name	dosage	container	no issued	date issued	issued to whom	tablets remaining	empty blister strips	dosage instructions	location
Temazepam	5mg	Box	60	19/2/03	deceased	4	56	2 nocté	bedside table
venlafaxine	75mg	Box	28	28/1/03	deceased	2	26	1 tds	kitchen cupboard

APPENDIX 5

Sample covering letter to send out with a draft statement

Dear

Further to our conversation on the telephone on .... I have typed up a statement and enclose this for you to read, amend and make additions as necessary. Please sign where indicated; please complete your occupation field and date with the date you sign the statement. I will make any necessary amendments to the statement before it is passed to the Coroner.

I enclose an addressed pre-paid envelope to return the statement to me.

Any queries please contact me on the above number.

Yours sincerely,

APPENDIX 6

Sample information request letter
(items requested will be tailored according to the circumstances of the death)

Dear

I write in connection with the death of *(deceased's name)* :

As you are aware from our previous telephone conversations, there will need to be an inquest into deceased's death and the Coroner will need to have some information from you about *him/her/deceased.*

I thought that if I were to ask you to write a letter to the Coroner with the information that he needs, such a course of action would give you time to think about your answers and write your reply in the way you want to. This might be preferable to me taking the information from you over the telephone – which can be a distressing process for some.

However if you would prefer that I talk you through the information on the telephone – please do not hesitate to ring me and I will of course go through that process with you.

Assuming that you would like to write a letter, please address it to *insert Coroner's details* and send it to *insert address.*

Please include the following information: *(this will vary according to the type of death)*
- The fact that *deceased* was your *specify relationship*, where *he/she* was born, and *his/her* date of birth
- The fact that deceased lived with *specify or lived alone* at address and how long *he/she* had lived there
- What sort of personality *deceased* had and what *his/her* interests were

- Whether *deceased* had any medical problems; if so, what was being done for *him/her* by *his/her* GP or by anyone else that you know about and whether you think this was helping *deceased* or not
- How often you saw *deceased*
- When you last saw *deceased*
- When you last spoke to *deceased* on the telephone (if this was later than when you last saw *him/her*)
- Anything particular that you can think of that might have caused *deceased* mental distress
- If you think *deceased* has taken *his/her* own life – and if so – why you think has done so
- If you think *deceased* has not taken *his/her* own life – why you think this
- Whether *deceased* talked about taking *his/her* life at any stage, and whether *he/she* had attempted to do so in the past
- Whether you have found or received any notes or messages from *deceased* since death

Please include any other information think that may be relevant but that I have not asked about

Thank you in advance for your help in this matter. I look forward to receiving your response in due course. The Coroner will then decide whether he will need you to be present at the inquest or not. (You should have received the leaflets I sent you in the post by now explaining about inquests. If not, please contact me.)

I enclose a reply paid envelope for your reply.

If you have any questions please do not hesitate to contact me

Yours sincerely

APPENDIX 7

Height Conversion

Metres & Cm	Feet & Inches	Metres & Cm	Feet & Inches
1.24	4′ 01″	1.78	5′ 10″
1.27	4′ 02″	1.80	5′ 11″
1.29	4′ 03″	1.83	6′ 00″
1.32	4′ 04″	1.85	6′ 01″
1.35	4′ 05″	1.88	6′ 02″
1.37	4′ 06″	1.90	6′ 03″
1.40	4′ 07″	1.93	6′ 04″
1.42	4′ 08″	1.95	6′ 05″
1.45	4′ 09″	1.98	6′ 06″
1.47	4 10″	2.01	6′ 07″
1.50	4 11″	2.03	6′ 08″
1.52	5′ 00″	2.06	6′ 09″
1.55	5′ 01″	2.08	6′ 10″
1.57	5′ 02″	2.11	6′ 11″
1.60	5′ 03″	2.13	7′ 00″
1.62	5′ 04″	2.16	7′ 01″
1.65	5′ 05″	2.18	7′ 02″
1.68	5′ 06″	2.21	7′ 03″
1.70	5′ 07″	2.23	7′ 04″
1.73	5′ 08″	2.26	7′ 05″
1.75	5′ 09″	2.28	7′ 06″

Weight Conversion

KGs	Total lbs	Stone	Pounds	KGs	Total lbs	Stone	Pounds
45.0	099	07	01	68.2	150	10	10
45.5	100	07	02	68.6	151	10	11
45.9	101	07	03	69.1	152	10	12
46.6	102	07	04	69.5	153	10	13
46.8	103	07	05	70.0	154	11	00
47.3	104	07	06	70.5	155	11	01
47.7	105	07	07	70.9	156	11	02
48.2	106	07	08	71.4	157	11	03
48.6	107	07	09	71.8	158	11	04
49.1	108	07	10	72.3	159	11	05
49.5	109	07	11	72.7	160	11	06
50.0	110	07	12	73.2	161	11	07
50.5	111	07	13	73.6	162	11	08
50.9	112	08	00	74.1	163	11	09
51.4	113	08	01	74.5	164	11	10
51.8	114	08	02	75.0	165	11	11
52.3	115	08	03	75.5	166	11	12
52.7	116	08	04	75.9	167	11	13
53.2	117	08	05	76.3	168	12	00
53.6	118	08	06	76.8	169	12	01
54.1	119	08	07	77.3	170	12	02
54.5	120	08	08	77.7	171	12	03
55.0	121	08	09	78.2	172	12	04
55.5	122	08	10	78.6	173	12	05
55.9	123	08	11	79.1	174	12	06
56.4	124	08	12	79.5	175	12	07
56.8	125	08	13	80.0	176	12	08
57.3	126	09	00	80.5	177	12	09
57.7	127	09	01	80.9	178	12	10
58.2	128	09	02	81.4	179	12	11
58.6	129	09	03	81.8	180	12	12
59.1	130	09	04	82.3	181	12	13
59.5	131	09	05	82.7	182	13	00
60.0	132	09	06	83.2	183	13	01
60.5	133	09	07	83.6	184	13	02
60.9	134	09	08	84.1	185	13	03
61.4	135	09	09	84.5	186	13	04
61.8	136	09	10	85.0	187	13	05
62.3	137	09	11	85.5	188	13	06
62.7	138	09	12	85.9	18	13	07
63.2	139	09	13	86.4	190	13	08
63.6	140	10	00	86.8	191	13	09
64.1	141	10	01	87.3	192	13	10
64.5	142	10	02	87.7	193	13	11
65.0	143	10	03	88.2	194	13	12
65.5	144	10	04	88.6	195	13	13
65.9	145	10	05	89.1	196	14	00
66.4	146	10	06	89.5	197	14	01
66.8	147	10	07	90.0	198	14	02
67.3	148	10	08	90.5	199	14	03
67.7	149	10	09	90.9	200	14	04

BMI chart

The Body Mass Index (BMI) is a tool that can be used to tell how healthy a person's weight is. If the height and weight are known, the BMI can be established:

Take the weight in kilograms (kg) and divide it by the height in metres (m); then divide the result by the height in metres again.

$$\textbf{Body mass index (BMI)} = \frac{\text{weight(kg)}}{\text{height(m)}2}$$

There are many internet sites offering an easy BMI calculator including www.nhsdirect.nhs.uk

Some pathologists now record BMI on post mortem examination reports

Underweight	Normal	Overweight	Obese	Morbidly obese
<18.4	18.4 – 24.9	25 – 29.9	30 – 39.9	>40

		XS		S		M		L		XL
US size		4	6	8	10	12	14	16	18	20
UK size		8	10	12	14	14/16	16	18	20	22
Chest / Bust	Ins	33	34	35	36	37	39	40	42	44
	Cms	84-85	86-88	89-90	91-94	95-98	99-102	103-107	108-112	113-117
Waist	Ins	25	26	27	28	29	31	32	34	36
	Cms	63-65	66-67	68-70	71-73	74-77	78-81	82-86	87-91	92-96
Hips	Ins	35	36	37	38	40	41	43	45	47
	Cms	90-91	92-94	95-96	97-100	101-104	105-108	109-113	114-118	119-123

Shoe sizes

EUR	UK		EUR	UK
35	3		42	8
36	3		43	9
37	4		44	10
38	5		45	11
39	6		46	11
40	6		47	12
41	7		48	13

Liquid volume:

To convert	Multiply by	
Imperial gallons to litres	4.55	1 gallon = 4.5 litres
Litres to imperial gallons	0.22	1 litre = .22 gallon
US gallons to litre	3.8	1 US gallon = 3.8 litres
Litres to US gallons	0.26	1 litre = .26 US gallons
US gallons to imperial gallons	0.83	
Imperial gallons to US gallons	1.20	

Distance:

To convert	Multiply by	
Inches to cms	2.54	1 inch = 2.54 cms
Cms to inches	0.39	1 cm = .39 inch
Feet to metres	0.30	1 ft = .30m
Metres to feet	3.28	1m = 3.28 ft
Yards to metres	0.91	1 yard = .91 metre
Metres to yards	1.09	1 metre = 1.09 yards
Miles to kilometres	1.61	1 mile -= 1.6 km
Kilometres to miles	0.62	1 km = .62 mile

Weight:

To convert	Multiply by	
Ounces to grams	28.35	1 oz = 28.35gr
Grams to ounces	0.035	1gr = .035oz
Pounds to kilograms	0.45	1 lb = .4555kg
Kilograms to pounds	2.20	1kg = 2.2lb

Temperature

To convert Fahrenheit to Centigrade subtract 32 and multiply by 0.555

To convert Centigrade to Fahrenheit multiply by 1.8 and add 32
320F = 00C

(Note all figures include a certain amount of tolerance and Coroner's Investigators should be aware that scientific accuracy may take figures to more decimal places.)

APPENDIX 8

PHONETIC ALPHABET

A	Alpha	N	November
B	Bravo	O	Oscar
C	Charlie	P	Papa
D	Delta	Q	Quebec
E	Echo	R	Romeo
F	Foxtrot	S	Sierra
G	Golf	T	Tango
H	Hotel	U	Uniform
I	India	V	Victor
J	Juliet	W	Whisky
K	Kilo	X	X-ray
L	Lima	Y	Yankee
M	Mike	Z	Zulu

The above information can be found in many places but a useful website to visit for all phonetic alphabets is www.phoneticalphabet.com

APPENDIX 9

Sample Investigation Plan
Death of: insert deceased's names, date of birth, date of death

Action	Person doing (if delegated)	Date done
Meet with family of deceased		
Determine strategy and tactics		
Statements		
Obtain statements from all relevant family members		
Obtain statement from last person to see deceased		
Obtain statement from last person to speak to deceased		
Obtain statement from finder		
Do own statement		
Other organisations		
Ambulance		
Obtain ambulance report		
Obtain copies of taped recordings of calls to and from ambulance service if relevant		
Medical		
Obtain report from GP		
Obtain hospital notes		
Obtain report from psychiatrist		
Obtain report from key worker / CPN		
Obtain post mortem examination report and toxicology report		
Print off updated relevant NICE Guidelines		

Trusts		
Get internal report of any Trust involved		
Get worksheet, care plan, CPA, risk assessment if psychiatric trust involved		
Obtain Trust notes		
Care Homes		
Obtain most recent one or two CQC inspection reports on the home		
Get action plans, fall assessment sheets, Waterlow Score sheets, daily notes, incident reports, Accident books, drug charts etc as relevant		
Police		
Obtain statement from senior CID officer who attended scene as to reasons death was not considered to be suspicious		
Refer to police child protection team for consideration if they need to be involved		
Refer to police vulnerable adult unit (or similar) for consideration if they need to be involved		
Obtain all relevant police serials		
Obtain any other relevant police information		
Obtain all photographs		

APPENDIX 10

SAMPLE FALLS CHECKLIST

Checklist of things to consider when investigating a death involving or due to a fall. This is not a prescriptive or exhaustive list. This is as well as the information for all statements and the generic checklist

Was this fall witnessed?	Who by? Obtain full details and a statement as to what happened
History of previous falls?	When, how often, any previous fractures?
Admitted to hospital? X-rays/scans?	Obtain copy x-ray or scan reports
Any disturbance of gait, mobility, muscle weakness?	Describe how this affected their walking / movement
What was the level of mobility?	
Did they use any mobility aids? Provide details	Eg Zimmer frame/crutches/ wheelchair/stick(s)
Any history of vertigo, inner ear problems, dizziness?	How long had this been going on? Was it being treated? With what?
Any cardiac history eg arrhythmias?	How long had this been going on? Was it being treated? With what?
Any evidence of osteoporosis/other related pathology?	
Any visual impairment?	Were spectacles worn? For long distance or close up? Were they being worn at the time of the fall?
Any cognitive impairment?	Describe fully
Any medication, outstanding or recent that may have contributed to likelihood to fall?	
On warfarin / similar? (See sep checklist.)	
What was their continence state?	Might urinary urgency or regular diarrhoea caused them to be hurrying?
Any known hazards in the house?	Eg too much furniture? Pets?
Were there any steps or stairs?	If so how many in the flight? What state of repair? Were they of uneven height and width? What state of repair were they in?

Was any footwear being worn at the time of the fall? If none were there bare feet or socks/ stockings	
What footwear was being worn?	Eg shoes / slippers / stockinged feet
What was the state of any footwear?	Were the shoes / slippers new with shiny and slippery soles? Or were they very old and worn with holes in the soles?
Were any steps or stairs involved in the fall?	Describe fully with width and height of each tread and riser especially noting if they were of equal height or uneven height
Was there any carpeting?	Describe the state of the carpeting eg threadbare, holes, loose
Any bedrails / cotsides? Any policy?	Obtain copy policy
Hip protection? Policy?	Obtain copy policy
What chair was being used? Any tray? What angle was it at?	
Any history of dementia/mental related factors?	
Any expressed fear of falling	
Was there any referral to a falls risk assessment service?	Provide full details with action taken
Obtain any relevant hospital notes	
Obtain a report from a medical practitioner	To cover all areas discussed above
Print off any relevant NICE guidelines	

APPENDIX 11

SAMPLE HEAD INJURY CHECKLIST

Checklist of things to consider when investigating a death involving or due to a head injury. This is not a prescriptive or exhaustive list. This is as well as the information for all statements and the generic checklist

What relevant PMH is there – eg epilepsy	Obtain copy of evidence Obtain report from GP
What co-pathologies were noted – eg alcohol /drugs	
What is the history immediately pre-injury?	
Who is this taken from? The patient themselves? If not from whom?	Obtain details of any other person providing information
How does this other know the information that is being given? Was this verified?	Obtain a statement from this person
What was the GCS score and at what stage?	
Did the GCS score change?	
What observations were done? How often? By whom?	
Where are the observation charts?	Obtain copies
Were there any changes? If so, what was done about them?	
What is the policy for dealing with head injuries?	Obtain copy
Was there a CT scan / MRI scan? If not why not?	If there was obtain copy any reports
What was done following any scan? Were the results received? By whom?	
What treatment was commenced post scan?	
Was there any consultation with a specialist neurological centre? Which centre? What consultation?	Obtain copy of evidence eg fax, email
When was the consultation? How?	Obtain name of doctor consulted
Obtain a copy of any 'Do not resuscitate' form	
Obtain copy relevant hospital notes	
Obtain copy NICE Guidelines	

APPENDIX 12

SAMPLE WARFARIN CHECKLIST

Checklist of things to consider when investigating a death involving the administration of Warfarin. This is not a prescriptive or exhaustive list. This is as well as the information for all statements and the generic checklist

What is the relevant past medical history? Eg atrial fibrillation, past DVT	Obtain a report from the GP
Why was this treatment being administered?	
When was it commenced?	
What checks have there been?	Eg regular blood tests
How often have the checks been?	
Where is the patient's INR card/record?	Obtain a copy
When was the INR level last checked?	
What is the past INR history?	Have their been previous bleeds/clots?
What is the most recent INR history?	
What is the INR level checking system?	Eg is the blood tested at the surgery/ home or sent to a hospital?
What is the system of notification to GP of blood test results?	Eg telephone call / fax / electronically?
What is the system of notification from the GP to the patient of blood test results?	Eg telephone call or visit by doctor or nurse
What action was taken once the results were received on the most recent occasion?	Who took the action? Get the name
Who was told about the most recent blood result? The patient themselves? Their carers?	
What arrangements were made to check INR level again; where & when?	
What questions were asked about symptoms eg bleeding?	
What is the doctor's/home's/hospital's Warfarin treatment policy?	Obtain a copy

APPENDIX 13

SAMPLE PRESSURE ULCERS CHECKLIST

Checklist of things to consider when investigating a death involving pressure sores. This is not a prescriptive or exhaustive list. This is as well as the information for all statements and the generic checklist

What is the relevant previous medical history?	Provide full information
What co-pathologies are there?	List fully
Did the patient have any acute, chronic or terminal disease which may have impacted on the inception or progression of pressure ulcers?	List fully
Was there any previous history of previous ulcers?	Obtain full details eg how long ago, what part of the body was affected
What was the patient's nutritional & hydration status?	Obtain copies food and hydration charts
What was the patient's cognitive status? Did this impact on the inception or progression of pressure ulcers?	
What was the patient's continence?	
Whereabouts on the body are the ulcers? Eg heels, sacrum, elbows, other	Specify location(s)
When did the ulcers arise?	
What grade were they? At what stage?	
What treatment was begun?	
Were tissue viability nurses involved in the treatment? If yes - who?	Obtain a statement from the tissue viability nurse(s)
What type of dressings were used? Who applied them?	Obtain details
Is there a Waterlow score assessment sheet?	Obtain any Waterlow score sheet
Was there any sensory impairment?	Obtain details
What was the assessment process?	
Was there a care plan involving regular turning and moving? Is there an accompanying 'moving" chart	Obtain copy plan and monitoring charts
Are there any charts / photographs?	Obtain copies

What special aids were provided? Eg ripple mattress? Was this on bed only or chair also?	
Were there any operations eg for debridement?	Obtain operation notes
Where is the care plan?	Obtain copy care plan
What policy?	Obtain copy policy
Obtain a report from the GP/ relevant consultant	To cover all above

APPENDIX 14

SAMPLE ASBESTOS RELATED DEATH CHECKLIST

Checklist of things to consider when investigating a death involving asbestos/ mesothelioma. This is not a prescriptive or exhaustive list. This is as well as the information for all statements and the generic checklist

List all known past employers	Names and addresses
Record the dates working for each employer as accurately as possible	Obtain copies of any documents that may show occupation and dates
What was the job title with each employer?	
What did that role involve exactly?	Provide as much detail as possible
Specifically – did they work with asbestos/ asbestos products	
What exactly did they do with it – eg paint it, cut it up, mould it	
Did the deceased know, before they died, of the likely diagnosis?	
If so, what did they say about their past jobs? Did they pick out any particular time, employer when they can say they were definitely in contact with asbestos	
What were their hobbies? Specifically - did any of those hobbies involve asbestos	
Remember to state the negative as well as the positives	eg – "he said before he died that he never worked with asbestos"
When did they show signs of illness?	
How was their health affected?	
Was there an "in life biopsy"; were there any pleural taps? Was the fluid sent for cytology? Was there pleuradesis?	Note the witness may not know this and you may get this information from the consultant, GP or hospital notes. However the witness may know
Has there been any process while the person was alive to apply for disablement benefit due to industrial disease?	If so, obtain copies of any documents possible re award of disablement benefit
Was any compensation awarded?	
Obtain details of any solicitors already involved	Contact solicitors for full information available

Has there been any process while the person was alive to sue any company for compensation?	If so, obtain copies of any documents possible re compensation or civil suit
Was any compensation awarded?	
Obtain details of any solicitors already involved	Contact solicitors for full information available
Offer the family a list of solicitors and leaflets re mesothelioma and details of website addresses	

REFERENCES

Published works

Davis, G; Lindsey, R; Seabourne, G; and Griffiths-Baker, J (2002) *Experiencing Inquests* HO Research Study 241   pub The Home Office Research, Development & Statistics Directorate ISBN 1 84082 903 6

Dorries, CP (1999) *Coroners' Courts: A Guide to Law and Practice.* Chichester. John Wiley

Dorries, CP (2004) *Coroners' Courts: A Guide to Law and Practice.* 2nd Edition Oxford

Matthews P (2002) *Jervis on the Office and Duties of Coroners: with forms and precedents* 12th ed. London: Sweet & Maxwell Ltd ISBN 0-421-78010-X

Knight, B. (1998) *Lawyer's Guide to Forensic Medicine* Cavendish Publishing ISBN 1859411592

Saukko, P.; Knight, B. (2004) *Knight's Forensic Pathology Third Edition.* London. Arnold ISBN 0340 76044 3

Slapper G (2003) *Legal errors, judicial inquiries, police numbers, coroners, lawyers and witnesses* Student Law Review 40: 23-26

Stone, G. (1999) *Suicide and Attempted Suicide* Carroll & Graf New York ISBN 0-7867-0940-5

Thomas, L; Friedman, D; Christian, L (2002) *Inquests: A practitioner's guide* LAG ISBN 0-905099-97-4

Statutes and Statutory Instruments

Asylum and Immigration Appeals Act 1993

Care Homes Regulations 2001 SI 3965

Children Act 2004

Coroners Act 1751

Coroners Act 1836

Coroners Act 1887

Coroners Act 1927

Coroners Act 1980

Coroners Act 1988

Coroners (Amendment) Rules 2005 SI 420

Coroners (Amendment) Rules 2008 SI 1652

Coroners and Justice Bill (laid before Parliament on 14/1/2009)

Coroners and Justice Act 2009 (due to receive Royal Assent October 2009)

Coroner's Rules 1984 SI 552

Corporate Manslaughter and Corporate Homicide Act 2007

Criminal Justice Act 1967

Criminal Justice and Public Order Act 1994

Criminal Procedure and Investigations Act 1996

Criminal Procedure and Investigations Act 1996 (Code of Practice) 2005 SI 985

Data Protection Act 1998

Health and Safety at Work etc Act 1974

Health and Social Care Act 2008

Human Rights Act 1988 (including European Convention on Human Rights)

Human Tissue Act 2004

Immigration Act 1971

Imprisonment (Temporary Provisions) Act 1980

Mental Health Act 1983

Misuse of Drugs Act 1971

National Clinical Assessment Authority (Establishment and Constitution) Amendment Order 2004

National Health Service and Community Care Act 1990

Police and Criminal Evidence Act 1984

Police Reform Act 2002

Railways and Transport Safety Act 2003

Railway Regulation Act 1842

Road Safety Act 2006

Road Traffic Act 1988

Road Traffic Act 1991

Suicide Act 1961

The Local Safeguarding Children Boards Regulations 2006 SI 90

The Social Security (Industrial Injuries) (Prescribed Diseases) Regulations 1985 SI 967

Stated cases

R v H M Coroner for North Humberside ex parte Jamieson (1995) QB1; 1994 3 All ER 972 and (1994) 3 WLR 82

R v Bristol Coroner ex parte Kerr (1974) 1 QB652; (1974) All ER 719

R v. Secretary of State for the Home Department (ex parte Amin) (2003) HL [2003] UKHL 51

Reports and Inquiries

Third Report Death Certification and the Investigation of deaths by Coroners The Shipman Inquiry July 2003 Cm5854

Death Certification and Investigation in England, Wales and Northern Ireland The Report of a Fundamental Review 2003 Cm 5831 TSO

Reforming the Coroner and Death Certification Service A Position Paper (March 2004) Home Office London Cm6159

The Report on the Provision of Coroner's Officers (2002) Home Office London

The Stephen Lawrence Inquiry (1999) Cm4262-1 TSO

Other works

Work-Related Deaths: A Protocol for Liaison (2003) The Health and Safety Executive MISC491 02/03 C140

FSID documents

Sudden unexpected deaths in infancy: A suggested approach for police and Coroner's Officers (2002) FSID

Recommendations for a joint agency protocol for the management of sudden unexpected deaths in infancy (2008) FSID

Health related documents

Information to the Coroner CMO Update 20/98 (1998) DH London

Cubicle rail suspension system with load release support systems (2002) NHS Estates London

Care Homes for Older People: National Minimum Standards (2003) Department of Health

Bed cubicle rails, shower curtain rails and curtain rails in psychiatric in-patients settings (2004) NHS Estates London

When a patient Dies: Advice on Developing Bereavement Services (2005) Department of Health, Human Tissue Branch, Bereavement Policy Gateway Ref 5578

Coroner Reform: The Government's Draft Bill Improving death investigation in England and Wales (2006) Cm 6849 TSO

Consultation on Improving the Process of Death Certification (2007) DH Leeds

Standards for Medium Secure Units: Quality Network for Medium Secure Units (2007) Royal College of Psychiatrists London

Why Children Die: A Pilot Study (2006) The Confidential Enquiry into Maternal and Child Health (2008)

Carbon monoxide: Are you at risk? (2008) (CWP) Produced by COI for the Department of Health

Improving the Process of Death Certification in England and Wales: Overview of Programme (2008) DH Leeds

Registering with the Care Quality Commission in relation to healthcare associated infection: Guidance for trusts 2009/10 (2008) CQC London

MHRA Medicines and Medical Devices Regulation: What you need to know (2008) London MHRA

Home Office documents

Deaths in Police Custody: Deaths of Members of the Public during or following Police Contact (2002) Home Office Circular 13/2002

Deaths in Police Custody: Guidance to the Police on Pre-Inquest Disclosure (2002) Home Office Circular 31/2002

Guide to Enforcement Interviewing (undated) Operational Enforcement Activity Chapter 42 UK Border Agency

MoJ documents

Coroner Reform and Additional Medical Advice A Discussion Document (2007) MoJ London

Statutory Duty for Doctors and other Public Service Personnel to Report Deaths to the Coroner (2007) MoJ London

Survey of the duties and practices of Coroner's Officers and administrative staff in England and Wales (2008) Ministry of Justice London

NICE documents

Infection control Prevention of healthcare-associated infections in primary and community care (2003) CG 2 Developed by Thames Valley University under the auspices of the National Collaborating Centre for Nursing and Supportive Care NICE London

Prevention of healthcare-associated infections in primary and community care Understanding NICE guidance – information for patients, their carers and the public (2003) NICE London

Self-harm: the short term physical and psychological management and secondary prevention of self-harm in primary and secondary care (2004) CG 16 Developed by the National Collaborating Centre for Mental Health NICE London

Self-harm: short-term treatment and management Understanding NICE guidance – information for people who self-harm, their advocates and carers, and the public (including information for young people under 16 years) (2004) Information from Clinical Guideline 16 NICE London

Falls: The assessment and prevention of falls in older people (2004) CG21 Developed by the National Collaborating Centre for Nursing and Supportive Care London

Falls: the assessment and prevention of falls in older people Understanding NICE guidance – information for older people, their families and carers, and the public Information about NICE clinical guideline 21 (2004) NICE London

The management of pressure ulcers in primary and secondary care: A Clinical Practice Guideline (2005) CG 29 Royal College of Nursing and National Institute for Health and Clinical Excellence London

Pressure ulcers prevention and treatment Understanding NICE guidance – information for people with pressure ulcers (also known as pressure sores or bed sores) and those at risk of developing pressure ulcers, their families and carers, and the public Information about NICE clinical guideline 29 (2005) NICE London

Atrial Fibrillation National clinical guidance for management in primary and secondary care (2006) CG 36 Royal College of Physicians London

Atrial Fibrillation: Information about NICE clinical guideline 36 (2006) NICE London

Head injury: Triage, assess ment, investigation and early management of head injury in infants, children and adults (2007) CG 56 Developed by the National Collaborating Centre for Acute Care London

The early management of head injuries: Information about NICE clinical guideline 56. (2007) NICE London

A guide to NICE (2005) NICE London

Multi-agency documents

Sudden Unexpected Death in Infancy: A Multi-Agency Protocol for Care and Investigation The report of a working group convened by the Royal College of Pathologists and the Royal College of Paediatrics and Child Health (2004) Royal College of Pathologists and the Royal College of Paediatrics and Child Health

Memorandum of Understanding: Investigating patient safety incidents involving unexpected death or serious untoward harm: a protocol for liaison and effective communications between the National Health Service, Association of Chief Police Officers and Health & Safety Executive (2006) Association of Chief Police Officers, Department of Health and Health and Safety Executive

Memorandum of Understanding agreed between the Rail Accident Investigation Branch, the British Transport Police, Association of Chief Police Officers and the

Office of Rail Regulation for the Investigation of Rail Accidents and Incidents in England And Wales (2006)

Memorandum of Understanding between the Coroners' Society of England and Wales and the Office of Rail Regulation (2008)

Memorandum of Understanding between the Coroners Society of England and Wales and Health and Safety Executive (2007) CSEW & HSE

Memorandum of Understanding between Royal National Lifeboat Institution and The Association of Chief Police Officers - Recovery of bodies from the water (2009) final draft ACPO

NPSA documents

Never Events Framework 2009/10 Process and Action for Primary Care Trusts 2009/10 (2009) NPSA NRLS London

Standardising wristbands improves patient safety Safer Practice Notice 24, (2007) NPSA London

Patient safety alert WHO Surgical Safety Checklist (2009) NPSA London

Patient safety alert Potassium chloride concentrate solutions, 2002 (updated 2003) NPSA London

Patient safety alert Reducing harm caused by misplaced nasogastric feeding tubes, (2005) NPSA London

Police documents

A Practical Guide to Investigative Interviewing (2000) National Police Training National Crime Faculty

ACPO Murder Investigation Manual (1988) & (2000)

Emergency Procedures Manual (2004) ACPO

Practical Guide to Investigative Interviewing (2004) Centrex (Central Police Training and Development Authority)

Road Death Investigation Manual V2 (2004) pub Centrex

Guidance on the management and recording and investigation of missing persons (2005) Produced on behalf of the Association of Chief Police Officers by the National Centre for Policing Excellence ACPO Centrex Hampshire

Guidance on the Use of Handcuffs (2006) ACPO London

Guidance on the Use of Incapacitant Spray (2006) ACPO London

Guidance on the Use of Limb Restraints (2006) ACPO London

Road Death Investigation Manual (2007) Produced on behalf of the Association of Chief Police Officers by the National Policing Improvement Agency

Investigative Interviewing Policy v1.3 (2007) Gloucestershire Constabulary

The Bureau Newsletter issue 1 September 2008 NPIA Hampshire

The Bureau Newsletter issue 3 April 2009 NPIA Hampshire

Transport related documents

The Investigation of Accidents or Serious Incidents to Public Transport Aircraft (undated) AAIB

The Investigation of Accidents to General Aviation Aircraft (undated) AAIB

GLOSSARY

ACPO	Association of Chief Police Officers
AAIB	Air Accident Investigation Board
ACCT	Assessment Care in Custody and Teamwork
AvMA	Action against Medical Accidents
BAFO	British Association of Forensic Odontologists
BCD	Buoyancy Control Device
BTP	British Transport Police
BTPA	British Transport Police Authority
BTPF	British Transport Police Force
CAB	Citizens Advice Bureaux
CBC	Child Bereavement Charity
CCTV	Close Circuit TeleVision
CEMACH	Confidential Enquiry into Maternal and Child Health
CHAI	Commission for Health and Audit Inspection
CHI	Commission for Health Improvement
CI	Coroner's Investigator
CID	Criminal Investigation Department
CIU	Collision Investigation Unit (or Crash Investigation Unit)
CJA	Criminal Justice Act
CJD	Creutzfeldt Jakob Disease
CMO	Chief Medical Office
CO	Carbon Monoxide
CO	Coroner's Officer
COA	Coroners' Officers Association
CPIA	Criminal Procedure and Investigation Act
CPN	Community Psychiatric Nurse
CPS	Crown Prosecution Service
CQC	Care Quality Commission
CRS	Coastguard Rescue Service
CRT	Coastguard Rescue Team
CSCI	Commission for Social Care Inspection
CSEW	Coroners Society of England and Wales

DH	Department of Health
DNA	Deoxyribonucleic acid
DoH	Department of Health
DoT	Department of Transport
DPB	Dental Practice Board
DPP	Director of Public Prosecutions
DVI	Disaster Victim Identification
ECHR	European Court of Human Rights
ECRI	Emergency Care Research Institute
EMI	Elderly Mentally Infirm
ESDA	Electrostatic Detection Apparatus
FCIRU	Forensic Collision Investigation and Reconstruction Unit
F&CO	Foreign and Commonwealth Office
FICO	Forensic Investigator Coroner's Officer
FLO	Family Liaison Officer
FSID	Foundation for the Study of Infant Deaths
FSS	Forensic Science Service
Fundamental Review	Death Certification and Investigation in England, Wales and Northern Ireland The Report of a Fundamental Review
GCS	Glasgow Coma Scale
GDC	General Dental Council
GMC	General Medical Council
GP	General Practitioner
HCAI	Health Care Association Infection
HIV	Human Immunodeficiency Virus
HM Coroner	Her Majesty's Coroner
HMCG	Her Majesty's CoastGuard
HO	Home Office
HOWP	Home Office Working Party
HRA	Human Rights Act
HSE	Health and Safety Executive
ICAS	Independent Complaints Advocacy Service
INR	International Normalised Ratio
IPCC	Independent Police Complaints Commission
IV	Intravenous

LA	Local Authority
LCD	Lord Chancellor's Department
LGA	Local Government Association
LSCB	Local Safeguarding Children Board
MAIB	Marine Accident Investigation Board
MCA	Magistrates' Courts Act
MCA	Marine and Coastguard Agency
MCCD	Medical Certificate as to Cause of Death
ME	Medical Examiner
MEO	Medical Examiner's Officer
MHAC	Mental Health Act Commission
MHRA	Medicine and Healthcare products Regulatory Agency
MICO	Medical Investigator Coroner's Officer
MoJ	Ministry of Justice
MoU	Memorandum of Understanding
MP	Member of Parliament
NBS	National Blood Service
NCAS	National Clinical Assessment Service
NCSC	National Care Standards Commission
NDPB	Non-Departmental Public Body
NEMA	National Emergency Mortuary Arrangements
NICE	National Institute for Health and Clinical Excellence
NHS	National Health Service
NHS BSA DSD	National Health Service Business Service Authority Dental Service Division
NHSLA	National Health Service Litigation Authority
NMC	Nursing and Midwifery Council
NMS	National Minimum Standards
NPIA	National Policing Improvement Agency
NPIA MPB	National Policing Improvement Agency Missing Persons Bureau
NPSA	National Patients Safety Agency
NRLS	National Reporting and Learning System
OFSTED	OFfice for STandards in Education,
ONS	Office for National Statistics
ORR	Office of Rail Regulation
PACE	Police and Criminal Evidence Act

PADI	Professional Association of Diving Instructors
PALS	Patient Advice and Liaison Service
PCT	Primary Care Trust
PEACE	Preparation and Planning; Engage and Explain; Account; Clarification and Challenge; Closure; Evaluation
PIR	Pre-Inquest Review
PM	Post mortem
PMH	Past Medical History
PNC	Police National Computer
PPO	Prisons and Probation Ombudsman
PSD	Professional Standards Department
RAIB	Rail Accident Investigation Board
RCPath	Royal College of Pathologists
RIDDOR	Reporting of Injuries, Diseases and Dangerous Occurrences Regulations
RLSS	Royal Life Saving Society
RMO	Registered Medical Officer
RNLI	Royal National Lifeboat Institution
ROSPA	Royal Society for Prevention of Accidents
RTA	Road Traffic Act
RTC	Road Traffic Collision
SAR	Search and Rescue
SCUBA	Self Contained Underwater Breathing Apparatus
SEAP	South East Advocacy Projects
SIO	Senior Investigating Officer
SLA	Service Level Agreement
SOBS	Survivors of Bereavement by Suicide
SOP	Standard Operating Procedure
SRA	Strategic Rail Authority
SUDI	Sudden Unexplained Death in Infancy
SUI	Serious Untoward Incident
TRL	Transport Research Laboratory
vCJD	new variant Creutzfeldt Jakob Disease
VSS	Victim Support Services
WHO	World Health Organisation

INDEX

Carboxyhaemoglobin	4.04.1.5
CEMACH	5.07.3
Checklist	2.01, 10.02.5, 11.02.6, Appendices 3, 10 - 14
Cherry pink	4.04.1.5
Child	
Child Bereavement Charity	5.07.1
Child deaths	5.01.2, 5.07
Choking	4.03.2, 4.03.3
CID	1.12.5, 1.16, 3.01.1, 17.03.3
Circumstances	2.07, 3.01, 4.01, 5.03, 5.05, 5.06
Cliffs	
Clothing	2.08, 3.01.4.4, 3.02.1, 3.02.2, 8.03, 8.03.4, 8.03.8, 13.05.4, 13.05.5, 14.03.2, 14.06
Coastguard	3.01.4, 3.02.2, 8.03.4, 8.03.10, 17.05
HMCG	3.02.2, 8.03.11
MCA	3.03.13, 8.03.11
Coroner's Society	5.08.2, 16.01
CPS	1.08.2, 2.04, 5.08.2, 5.08.3, 5.08.7, 9.04.4
CQC	1.04.2, 6.0.5, 9.05.1, 9.08.2, 10.04.2, 11.02.7, 12.02.6
Cyanosis	4.03
Deceased	2.03, 3.01, 3.03, 4.01, 5.02, 5.03, 5.04, 5.05, 5.06
Decomposed	1.09.3, 14.04.1, 14.04.4, 14.05.1, 14.05.3.1
Dental	1.04.2, 6.05, 8.03.8, 8.03.9, 9.05.4, 10.01, 14.03.1, 14.04.1, 14.05.1, 14.05.3.1, 14.05.4.1, 14.06
Diagnosis	4.03.3.1, 5.06.2, 10.02.4.1, 10.03.1.1, 11.02.5.1, 17.02.1,
Dignitas	4.05
Disasters	1.16
Dive	3.01.4.9, 3.03
DNA	14.06
Downgrading	1.15
Drowning	1.10.2, 1.12.6, 3.01.4.3, 3.01.4.4, 3.01.5, 3.02, 3.03, 3.03.5, 5.04.8, 17.04
dry-lung	3.01.3
Wet	3.01.2
Drug	1.12.2, 1.12.4, 2.03, 3.01.4.1, 3.01.4.12, 3.03.2, 4.01.10, 4.03.3.2, 4.03.4, 5.02.4, 5.05.2, 6.02.3.1, 6.02.3.2, 7.01.2.1, 7.01.2.5, 7.02, 8.01.2.7, 8.02.2.5, 8.03.7, 8.30.8, 8.03.9, 9.07.1, 9.07.2, 9.08.2, 10.02.4.1, 10.02.4.2, 10.03.1.1, 10.03.1.3, 10.04, 10.04.1.1, 11.02.5.1, 11.02.5.2, 11.02.6, 11.03.6.2, 12.02.5, 13.09.3, 16.03, Appendix 4

Electrical deaths	5.06
Emergency mortuary	1.16
Event	2.08, 3.01, 3.03, 4.01, 5.02, 5.03, 5.04, 5.05, 5.06
Evidence	1.03, 1.05, 1.07.1, 1.08, 1.08.1, 1.08.2, 1.08.5.2, 1.08.5.4, 1.09.4, 1.09.6, 1.10.2, 1.12.1, 1.12.2, 1.12.3, 1.12.4, 1.13.1, 1.15.1, 1.15.1.2, 1.15.2, 1.15.3.2, 1.15.3.3, 1.16, 2.02, 2.04, 2.05, 2.10, 2.11, 3.01.3, 3.01.4.11, 3.03, 3.03.2, 4.01.9, 4.01.11, 4.02.1, 4.03.3.1, 4.04.1.7, 4.04.1.7, 4.04.2.4, 4.05, 5.01.1, 5.02.1, 5.02.2, 5.02.6, 5.04.7, 5.05.4, 5.05.5, 5.05.9, 5.06.7, 5.08.2, 5.09, 6.02.3.10, 6.03.1, 6.03.5.9, 7.01.2.1, 7.01.2.3, 7.02.1.2, 7.02.1.5, 702.10, 7.02.2.2, 7.02.2.5, 7.02.2.7, 7.03.5, 8.01.2.8, 8.02.2.1, 8.02.2.5, 8.03.9, 9.04.1, 9.04.4, 9.05.6, 9.07.1, 9.08.1, 13.02.2, 13.04, 13.05.1, 13.05.2, 13.06, 13.06.1, 13.07, 13.08.2, 13.09.9, 13.09.10, 14.02, 14.03.1, 14.03.2, 14.04.1, 14.05.3.1, 14.05.3.2, 14.05.3.3, 15.02, 15.03.4, 15.03.5, 15.05.1, 16.03, 16.06, 16.04, 17.03.1, 17.03.3.7, 17.04
Gatherin/ seizure	1.08.4, 1.08.5.3, 1.09.5, 1.11, 1.12.6, 1.13.2, 2.10, 3.01.4.13, 4.01.11, 4.02.1, 5.06.7, 7.02.1.9, 7.02.2.12, 10.02.4.2, 10.03.1.3, 11.02.5.2, 11.03.6.2, 17.03.3.5, 17.03.4,
Exhaust	4.04.1.4, 4.04.1.6, 4.04.2.6
Exhibit	1.09.4, 2.06, 13.01, 13.05.5, 13.08.1, 13.10.1, 15.05, 16.03, 16.04,
Falls	2.05, 3.01.4.7, 7.01.2.1, 7.01.2.2, 7.02.2.6, 8.03.3, 9.06.1, 11.02.5.1, 11.03.5, 11.03.6.2, Appendix 10
FCO	5.09
Finder	2.04, 3.01, 3.03, 4.01, 4.04
Fingerprints	14.06
Fire	5.05
FLO	5.02
Forensic	
post mortem examination	1.13.3
Forensic Science Service	1.13.3.3, 5.05.1, 14.05.1
Friends at the end	4.05
FSID	5.07
Funeral Directors	15.03
Gases	
argon	4.05
butane	4.05